T0219562

#SocialMedia in #HealthCare

A Guide to Creating Your Professional Digital Presence

#SocialMedia in #HealthCare

A Guide to Creating Your Professional Digital Presence

Mona Shattell, PhD, RN, FAAN
Twitter: @MonaShattell
LinkedIn: Mona Shattell
Website: influence-rx.com

Melissa Batchelor, PhD, RN, FNP, FAAN
Twitter: @MelissaBPhD
Facebook Page: Melissa Batchelor
Instagram: @MelissaBPhD_TheNurse
LinkedIn: Melissa Batchelor
YouTube: MelissaBPhD
Website: MelissaBPhD.com

Rebecca Darmoc, MS
Twitter: @RebeccaDarmoc
LinkedIn: Rebecca Darmoc
Website: influence-rx.com

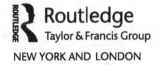
Routledge
Taylor & Francis Group

NEW YORK AND LONDON

First published 2022 by SLACK Incorporated

Published 2024 by Routledge
605 Third Avenue, New York, NY 10158

and by Routledge
4 Park Square, Milton Park, Abingdon, Oxon, OX14 4RN

Routledge is an imprint of the Taylor & Francis Group, an informa business

Library of Congress Cataloging-in-Publication Data

Names: Shattell, Mona, author.
Title: Social media in health care : a guide to creating your professional
   digital presence / Mona Shattell, PhD, RN, FAAN, Melissa Batchelor, PhD,
   RN, FNP, FAAN, Rebecca Darmoc, MS.
Description: Thorofare, NJ, USA : SLACK Incorporated, [2022] | Includes
   bibliographical references and index.
Identifiers: LCCN 2022010613 (print) | ISBN 9781630919092 (paperback) |
Subjects: LCSH: Social media in medicine. | Nurse and patient. | BISAC:
   COMPUTERS / Internet / Social Media | MEDICAL / Nursing / Reference
Classification: LCC R859.7.S63 S53 2022 (print) |
   DDC 610.285--dc23/eng/20220613
LC record available at https://lccn.loc.gov/2022010613

Cover Artist: Katherine Christie

ISBN: 9781630919092 (pbk)
ISBN: 9781003526452 (ebk)

DOI: 10.4324/9781003526452

Contents

ABOUT THE AUTHORS

Mona Shattell, PhD, RN, FAAN is Chair of the Department of Nursing Systems, Hugh F. and Jeannette G. McKean Endowed Chair, and Professor at the University of Central Florida in Orlando. She is the Editor of the *Journal of Psychosocial Nursing and Mental Health Services*, and the author of more than 150 journal articles and book chapters. Her published work focuses on patient-provider relationships, various environments of care, and underserved populations such as long-haul truckers. Dr. Shattell is a Fellow in the American Academy of Nursing. She is an active social media user, content developer, and public thought leader. She has published op-eds in the *New York Times*, *The Atlantic*, Health Affairs Blog, and others. She was named one of the "Top 25 Most Influential Nurses to Follow on Twitter" and is #4 on the list of "100 Twitter Feeds Every Nurse Should Follow." Prior to joining the faculty at UCF College of Nursing, she was the Associate Dean of Faculty Development and Professor at the Johns Hopkins School of Nursing; she served as Chair and Professor in the College of Nursing at Rush University; she served as Associate Dean for Research and Faculty Development and Professor in the College of Science and Health at DePaul University; Associate Professor at the University of North Carolina at Greensboro, Assistant Professor at the University of Alabama at Birmingham, and Lecturer at the University of North Carolina at Charlotte. Dr. Shattell received a PhD in nursing from the University of Tennessee Knoxville, a Master of Science degree in psychiatric mental health nursing from Syracuse University, and a Bachelor of Science degree in nursing, also from Syracuse University.

Melissa Batchelor, PhD, RN, FNP, FAAN is an Associate Professor at George Washington University School of Nursing and Director of the Center for Aging, Health and Humanities. She is a Fellow in the American Academy of Nursing and served the United States Senate Special Committee on Aging as a Health and Aging Policy Fellow. Her research focuses on improving mealtimes for those living with Alzheimer's disease by teaching caregivers to use three supportive handfeeding techniques. Dr. Batchelor is a nationally recognized innovator in using digital technology and social media. A family caregiving video series she co-developed with the AARP's Home Alone Alliance was a selected as a finalist for the 2020 Sharecare Awards—an award established by Sharecare and National Academy of Television Arts & Sciences, New York Chapter (renowned for the Emmy Awards). She has been invited to share her journey with social media through presentations for the National Academy of Medicine, Science, and Engineering and the American Academy of Nursing, among others. She was selected for the American Association of Colleges of Nursing's 2019 Digital Innovation Bootcamp and completed requirements to be an Apple Teacher. Her website MelissaBPhD.com houses her handfeeding demonstration videos and a television series produced by Fairfax County Public Access Television. In 2020 she started a weekly podcast called *This is Getting Old: Moving Towards an Age-Friendly World*. The podcasts are disseminated through YouTube, Facebook, Twitter, Instagram, and LinkedIn and can also be found on iTunes, Amazon Music, Spotify, and Stitcher. In the first year, the podcasts have 13,000 Subscribers on YouTube, more than 1 million viewing hours, 9 million impressions, and more than 8000 downloads from the podcast platforms.

Rebecca Darmoc, MS is the Chief Marketing Officer for a consulting firm and former director of marketing at Rush University System for Health, an academic medical system in Chicago. As a brand strategist, she actively coaches faculty, clinicians, and researchers on personal branding and public communications. With a master's degree in Integrated Marketing Communications from Northwestern University, she specializes in content marketing, persuasive messaging, and social influence. She is a member of the Forbes Communications Council and has specialty certificates in social media marketing, content marketing strategy, and leveraging neuroscience for business impact. She was named one of "10 Most Influential Women Leaders of 2021" by Industry Era magazine. Her work has been recognized by international content marketing associations with the Silver Pearl Award for Best Healthcare/Pharmaceutical Content 2017 and first place for Best University Publication 2018.

FOREWORD

Health care has changed drastically over the last several decades. Innovative medical discoveries, novel therapeutics, and digital innovation have been at the forefront of these exciting changes. With the rise of the internet and opportunities for global connectivity with multiple social media platforms, the delivery of health care and public health communications has also shifted. The responsibility of health care workers has always been to provide unbiased, evidence-based care to all who require medical care and provide education to not only their patients but also the communities they serve. Prior to the internet, communication with communities regarding public health messaging occurred predominantly in the clinic, through the newspaper or television, or in the community such as at the grocery store, in church, at family gatherings, or other community events and types of engagement. As social media has become a fixture in many lives, as well as a simple way to access a wealth of information, and an excellent way to engage in dialogue with many individuals from different backgrounds in a seamless manner, the strategies for public health communication have changed dramatically. Unfortunately, education on this type of engagement and public health communication or messaging have not yet been incorporated into medical curricula, and there is a real need to provide guidance and skills in this arena to health care professionals, from students to senior faculty and clinicians.

In the past, misconceptions or "old wives'" tales regarding home remedies and the pathophysiology of certain illnesses was typically passed within families and friends, but often did not take hold at a national level, with no fast and easy way to quickly disseminate the information. Health care workers were able to address these questions and concerns at clinic visits or in individual conversations, and medical care was able to be provided after acknowledging and addressing these questions. With the advent of the internet and social media, rapid dissemination of non–peer reviewed, and nonfactual information is done with ease, and often with a targeted strategic approach. For years the health care community was advised to avoid engaging in the online space to maintain a level of professionalism and prevent the blurring of the "doctor-patient relationship." Unfortunately, as the digital highway has become a pervasive aspect of most individuals' lives, by not engaging in these spaces health care workers are allowing others without medical backgrounds, who often are promoting messaging with some hope for personal gain, to drive the narrative and provide inaccurate information to the community. During the COVID-19 pandemic, this was amplified and resulted in an infodemic of massive proportions fueled by misinformation and disinformation that has cost countless numbers of lives. When individuals are using inaccurate, often dangerous, information they have found or heard about online, entire communities can be impacted.

Social Media in Health Care is a book that talks about the power of health care workers' voices being showcased on the international stage, and the utility of engaging in the social media space as a health care worker cannot be understated. For the messaging and strategies to be effective, health care workers need the knowledge and understanding of how to best engage and participate in the online space. This book provides an education on social media and engagement online for health care professionals that is not provided in traditional educational programs.

— *Shikha Jain, MD, FACP*
Assistant Professor of Medicine
Division of Hematology and Oncology
Director of Communication Strategies in Medicine
University of Illinois Chicago
Associate Director of Oncology Communication & Digital Innovation
University of Illinois Cancer Center
Chicago, Illinois

Twitter: @ShikhaJainMD
Instagram: @ShikhaJainMD
Website: www.shikhajainmd.com

INTRODUCTION

"Like all technology, social media is neutral but is best put to work in the service of building a better world."

Simon Mainwaring
@simonmainwaring

The path to influence and thought leadership has changed dramatically over the past decade. All types of mass communication, from the beginning of time, have had the same purpose—to educate, entertain, persuade, and influence public opinion. Now that we're in the "age of mobile," there has been a major shift in media influence—from corporate control to consumer control.

More Accessible Than Ever. As consumers, all we need is a digital device and Wi-Fi connection to publish our own content, ideas, and expert opinions online. We also reap the benefits of a society that is skeptical of corporate communications. Studies of consumers show that the overwhelming majority of people trust individuals more than brands—even if the consumers don't know the individuals. And online, we engage with people more than we engage with brands.

Beyond the Hospital Walls and Ivory Tower. This shift offers an opportunity for health care professionals. It allows us to articulate the meaning of our work and research beyond our institutions and beyond professional presentations and publications in peer-reviewed journals— anytime and anywhere. It allows us to connect with the public and specific patient communities to share our knowledge and expertise.

Social Media Is About Conversations. Your online presence gives you an instant line of communication to your peers and the public; people are online right now looking for experts, having conversations, and making connections. A professional online presence allows you to share your own knowledge with a much larger audience. You become a trusted source of information that brings value to others.

Path to Digital Influence. This book supports all engagement levels from health care students to seasoned professionals. It will take you through the Consume, Contribute, and Create model to help guide your journey. Whether you are a social media novice or have an established digital presence, our goal is to share proven ways that you can expand your influence and impact.

What to Expect. This book can be read from cover to cover or used as a reference when you want to learn about a specific aspect of social media or need an idea for what to share. This is a book on principles for using social media because the platforms can, and do, change all the time. These principles are the same and are effective for all professions, and you will adapt them to the social media platform that is best for your professional development. Although we share tactics and examples for the principles, the examples are not exhaustive as the digital world changes daily.

For more current, contextual examples for applying the principles, you can reference the influence-rx.com and MelissaBPhD.com websites, blogs, and podcasts.

Why Did We Write the Book? We have experienced success using technology and social media to do everything we recommend and teach you to do in this book—we have walked the walk that we base our talk on. We each had a natural interest in developing our own social media skills and our different experiences complemented each other. We wanted to share our collective strategies with other health care professionals to amplify accurate health care messages for the public. We wanted to help health care professionals, academics, and scientists expand their reach, build a community, and/or raise awareness about health-related content.

Disclaimer: Apple-Centric. The discussion and resources put forth in the book are primarily framed around Apple-based products because we use Macs, iPhones, and iPads. However, the principles we recommend are the same, whether it comes from the Apple App Store or you find the same or similar versions for your Android devices in Google Play.

Learn to Create Innovative Products

Educators. If you are an educator, you can build foundational skills to use Apple educational products using a Mac or iPad (e.g., iMovie, Keynote, Pages, and GarageBand), by becoming an Apple Teacher [free training] (Apple Inc., 2020). Visit the appleteacher.apple.com website to register and complete the first six badges from either the iPad or Mac Collection.

Non-Educators. If you are not an educator, Apple also offers free training sessions through the Today at Apple program. To find live, in-person sessions for training, use the Apple Store app to find "Sessions" based on your location. You can also find YouTube tutorial videos to learn to do anything else you find interesting.

REFERENCES

Apple Inc. (2020). *Apple Teacher*. https://apple.co/37CIHyW

Aselage, M. (2010). Mobilizing gerontological nursing education: The GNEC podcast project. *Journal of Gerontological Nursing, 36*(7), 63-64. https://doi.org/10.3928/00989134-20100527-01

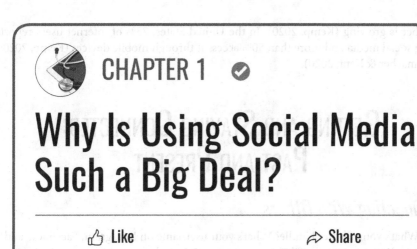

Why Is Using Social Media Such a Big Deal?

👍 **Like**　　　　　　　　　↪ **Share**

> "Content is fire, and social media is gasoline."
>
> *Jay Baer*
> *@JayBaer*

Why have a public voice? As health care professionals, it is our responsibility to be part of the conversations about health, illness, disease, prevention, research, and current topics in the news related to science. Many of these conversations are happening on social media and are part of our daily lives. Social media is ubiquitous, and you might already have an opinion formed on whether this is good or bad for our society. Although people can use social media to create discord or disruption, our goal is talk about the good it does for society; and how you, as health care professionals, can play a role.

BY THE NUMBERS

There are more than 4.5 billion people in the world who use the internet an average of more than 6.5 hours per day (Kemp, 2020). In the United States and other high-income countries, 90% or more of adults use the internet or own an internet-connected handheld device (i.e., smartphone, mobile device; Schumacher & Kent, 2020). Social media users are now at 3.8 billion people worldwide and that

Shattell, M., Batchelor, M., & Darmoc, R. *Social Media in Health Care: A Guide to Creating Your Professional Digital Presence* (pp. 1-23).

number is growing (Kemp, 2020). In the United States, 73% of internet users report using social media and more than 50% access it through mobile devices (Kemp, 2020; Schumacher & Kent, 2020).

Getting and Staying Connected: Past and Present

Connecting With Others

What's your Twitter handle? What's your username on Instagram, Facebook, and/or LinkedIn? Are you on TikTok or SnapChat? In today's world, you're much more likely to be asked for this information to connect personally and professionally rather than being asked for your business card with your phone number or email address. The world is now digital.

How We Get Our News Today

In the past, we relied on printed newspapers and television programs to get our news. As the world has become more digital, mass communication outlets have adapted. The number of Americans who get their news from social media continues to increase every year with 55% of U.S. adults reporting that they "often" or "sometimes" use social media to Consume the news (Shearer & Grieco, 2019).

Mainstream Media Meets Social Media

Local and national news programs and news anchors display their hashtags and handles on the television screen news ticker. Screenshots of tweets (the term for content delivered through the Twitter platform) from politicians, celebrities, and corporations are shared on morning, nightly, and cable news stations to "report" points of view, new policies, or crisis communications in real time. We can connect at any time of day, from anywhere, to follow news trends more easily than ever using social media.

What Exactly Is Social Media?

Platforms and Apps

Social media is roughly defined as a group of internet-based platforms and apps that allow the creation and exchange of user-generated content, which has added an online layer to our offline lives (Van Dijck, 2013). These platforms and apps influence human interaction at an individual, community, and societal level allowing unprecedented global connection and interaction. As individuals, all we need is a mobile device and WiFi connection to publish our own content, ideas, and expert opinions online. According to Merriam-Webster, social media is defined as "forms of electronic communication (such as websites for social networking and microblogging) through which users create online communities to share information, ideas, personal messages, and other content (such as videos)" (Merriam-Webster, n.d.).

HISTORY OF SOCIAL NETWORKING AND SOCIAL MEDIA

Where Did It All Start?

Let's take a minute to reflect on the history of social networking and the evolution of social media. Depending on how old you are, you may have lived through some of these socio-cultural experiences. Over the past 2 decades, social media has risen from being an activity only accessible to a few to being a global, daily experience for the majority of people (Table 1-1).

Social Networking

SixDegrees (1997) has been heralded as the first social networking site, allowing users to create a profile and "friend" other users, send and post messages, and create degrees of relationship closeness (e.g., first-, second-, third- degree), hence the name (Hendricks, 2019; McFadden, 2020). From these early beginnings, social networking and social media have evolved based on features users liked and are now social media "norms."

Profiles

Friendster (2002) was the first social networking site also used for dating and event announcements. Profiles were private and only visible to registered users, and it was the first to incorporate "status updates" to indicate your current mood and allowed you to message "friends of friends" (McFadden, 2020; Samur, 2018). Myspace (2003) was the first to allow users to completely customize their profiles that were visible to anyone (in contrast to Friendster) and allowed users to embed music and videos for the first time (Hendricks, 2019; McFadden, 2020).

Like or Unlike

Hot or Not (2000) was the beginning of users being able to submit a photograph in order to have others rank their level of attractiveness, a precursor to the "Like" or "Unlike" feature (Samur, 2018). Facebook (2005), described as Harvard's answer to Hot or Not, expanded the Like/Unlike features to include other options: Like, Love, Care, Haha, Wow, Sad, and Angry.

#Hashtags

The most significant contribution for social media has been the hashtag—a symbol used to organize and aggregate key words used in tweets, and most recently key words across most social media platforms (Hendricks, 2019; McFadden, 2020).

TABLE 1-1. HISTORICAL TIMELINE OF SOCIAL MEDIA

YEAR(S)	PLATFORM	
1997	SixDegrees	Users could upload a profile and "friend" other users. As the platform name indicates, users were able to send messages and post to bulletin boards to expand their social groups in first-, second-, third-degree (etc.) connections.
1998	Moveon.org	One of the first social activist websites. Began as an email chain passing around petitions to oppose President Bill Clinton's impeachment.
1999	LiveJournal and others	Emergence of blogging sites encouraged users to follow each other and create groups that interacted with one another. This form of social media is still popular today.
2000	Hot or Not	Users submitted photos and others could rate their attractiveness.
2000	LunarStorm	First commercial, advertisement-financed social networking site, with teenagers as the target audience.
2002	Friendster	Used for typical social networking but also served as a dating site and event, hobby, and concert discovery service. You could create a profile, include "status updates" to indicate your current mood, and message "friends of friends of friends." Profiles were private and only visible to registered users.
2002	LastFM	One of the first online music sites with music databases and online radio streaming services that are now commonplace.
2003	LinkedIn	Unique social media site focused on business.
2003	Myspace	First platform to allow users to completely customize their profile, embed music and videos. Profiles were visible to anyone, a contrast to Friendster.
2003	WordPress	Opened blogging and website development to a broader audience.

(continued)

Table 1-1. Historical Timeline of Social Media (continued)

YEAR(S)	PLATFORM	
2003	Photobucket Flickr	First sites to allow photosharing.
2003	The Facebook (2003 version was Facemash)	Described as Harvard's answer to Hot or Not. In 2005, after registering one million users, name changed to Facebook after domain name was purchased for $200K.
2005	YouTube	Launched an entirely new method of communication by allowing users to create and share media over very long distances.
2005	Reddit	Reddit is an American social news aggregation, web content rating, and discussion website. Registered members submit content to the site such as links, text posts, and images, which are then voted up or down by other members.
2006	Facebook	Advent of what many consider the beginning of social media—platform allows connection on the internet, and by extension, the world. In 2006, registration was opened up to everyone—going from an exclusive Harvard-only club to a global network.
2006	Twitter	Originally envisioned as a text message–based tool for sending updates between friends, Twitter now allows users to interact directly with international leaders, celebrities, businesses, and other consumers—a level of engagement previously unheard of. Twitter's strict 140-character limit for tweets set it apart from Facebook and Tumblr, although they increased the character limit to 280 in November 2017.
2009	Spotify Foursquare	Continued development of niche platforms—Spotify for music, podcasts, and other audio content; Foursquare was one of the first that allowed users to "check in" while sharing recommendations about their favorite neighborhoods and cities with family and friends.
2010	Instagram	Launch of Instagram—a U.S.-based photo and video sharing platform available on almost all smart device platforms and allows users to edit uploaded content within the app (exclusively) and organize material using tags and other location information. Instagram posts were the first to allow filters for photos.
2011	Snapchat	Launched as an app that enabled users to post photos/videos that disappeared from site after a few moments.
2016 to 2017	Musical.ly becomes TikTok	Musical.ly was the precursor app converted to a short-form video sharing app of lip syncing, comedy, and other niches such as health, fashion, business, pets, and even short films.

Adapted from Gayton C. (2020, July 18). *The origins of TikTok.* ChristinaGayton.medium.com. https://bit.ly/3uNlFxJ; Nguyen T. (2021, February 10). *Clubhouse, the invite-only audio app, explained.* Vox.com. https://bit.ly/3fOho9f; O'Connell B. (2020, February 28). *History of Snapchat: Timeline and facts.* TheStreet.com. https://bit.ly/3yUbrPD

Niche Platforms and Advances in Sharable Content

Niche platforms began to emerge as more social media platforms came on the market. Moveon.org was one of the first social activist websites (1998) and began as an email chain opposing President Bill Clinton's impeachment (McFadden, 2020). LinkedIn (2003) focuses only on business and continues to highlight first-, second-, and third-degree connections.

Blogs

Blogs made their debut through sites like LiveJournal (1999) but gained greater accessibility through the advent of WordPress (2003), which made it possible for anyone to create their own website with templates (McFadden, 2020; Shearer & Grieco, 2019).

Photos

Photobucket and Flickr (2003) were the first photo-sharing platforms. Instagram (2010) launched as a video and photo-sharing app specifically for mobile devices, that allowed users to upload image-based content exclusively within the app, and was the first to create filters for users to add to their photos (McFadden, 2020; Samur, 2018).

Videos

YouTube (2005) launched an entirely new method of communication for video-sharing, allowing users to communicate with a global audience by uploading, sharing, and viewing video content and tracking views and likes of that content. Within 1 year, YouTube was receiving 8 million views per day (McFadden, 2020).

Music

Spotify and Foursquare (2009) continued the development of niche platforms: Spotify for audio content (e.g., music, podcasts), and Foursquare was the first to allow users to "check in" to locations on a map while sharing recommendations about their favorite neighborhoods and cities with family and friends (Samur, 2018).

Local to Global Connection

Facebook started off as Facemash (2003) and registered one million users. In 2006, Facebook moved from being an exclusive Harvard-only club and changed over the next several years into a global network using the internet to connect users around the world (McFadden, 2020; Samur, 2018). Twitter (2006), originally envisioned as a text-only tool to send updates between friends, was the first to allow users to directly interact with international leaders, celebrities, and businesses through brief chats (or "micro-blogging" as it's called)—a level of engagement previously unheard of.

Computers to Mobile Devices

As technology and smartphones evolved, social media also evolved from being solely internet platform-based (computers) to app-based (mobile devices). Today, many platforms are available on both. For example, Twitter began online in 2006 and didn't develop its official mobile app until 2010 (Brown, 2019). As technology has advanced, social media has capitalized on each development over time and includes more and more features, driven by user response and demand, and new revenue models of technology companies.

Commercialization

The first commercialization of social media through advertisements began with LunarStorm (2000) and this has become a major market driver (McFadden, 2020). Today, the social media business model hinges on monetization of content and targeted ads based on user profiles (Gil, 2019). As "subscribers" to social media platforms, users provide their name, age, location, and other personal details, which allows marketers to use the data to learn what you like and who you know (Gil, 2019).

OTHER WAYS SOCIAL MEDIA HAS CHANGED THE WORLD

Language

Social media has a language of its own and if you're new to social media, learning the "social media language" is a critical first step (Table 1-2). Social media has become pervasive in modern society, and many of these words used are now being defined in traditional dictionaries. Words used in social media may or may not translate into their typical use.

Integration Into Culture

In the past, we used the word "tweet" as a noun ("the chirp of a young bird") and as a verb ("to make a chirping noise"). In 2013, the Oxford English Dictionary added another meaning for "tweet" as a noun to mean "a post made on the social media application Twitter" and as a verb "to make a post on the social media application Twitter" (Oxford English Dictionary, 2020). Other examples of social media terms have been integrated into today's culture include "mention" and "notification." One might "mention" a news event in conversation to "notify" you of the event, but "mention" in Twitter means someone includes your name in the body of a tweet to draw attention to you and a "notification" lets you know you have news or an update. Knowing the different terms related to social media is a first step in learning to talk the talk.

TABLE 1-2. SOCIAL MEDIA TERMS DEMYSTIFIED

TERM	DEFINITION	PLATFORM
Activity feed	Notifications of new followers, likes, and comments of posts.	Instagram
Algorithm	Mathematical rules that social media companies use to determine what content individuals see on their news feed and what ads show up on accounts based on previous online activity and behavior. Algorithms are also used by web browsers to send individuals targeted ads and rank search results.	Facebook Instagram LinkedIn Twitter Web
Animoji	A personalized or character emoji that copies the movements of your face and allows you to add an audio component to communication.	Text
App	Short for "application" or mobile app is a computer application that is downloaded onto a mobile device. Software program for mobile phones/tablets.	Mobile device or tablet versions of: Facebook Instagram LinkedIn Twitter
Bio	Part of the profile page, this section is the individual or organization's narrative descriptive information that allows concise differentiation among users.	Facebook Instagram LinkedIn Twitter Web
Bitmoji	A personalized cartoon emoji that can be used in online communication through platforms and text messages.	Text
Blog	A truncation of "weblog"; a blog is a discussion or informational website published on the internet with posts that are often informal diary-style written entries. The main purpose of a blog is to connect you with your audience and boost traffic to send quality leads to your professional website. Intended as more frequent, longer posts, blogs give you a higher chance of your website being found and discovered by your audience.	Web
Chat	Non-verbal real-time communication such as sending texts back and forth. Chats are intended to be short and enable participants to respond quickly, thereby giving a feeling similar to spoken conversation.	Text Twitter
Comment	A response provided as an answer, reaction, or opinion to a blog, message, or post on social media.	Facebook Instagram LinkedIn Twitter YouTube
Connecting	Connections made between people and organizations by clicking the "connect" button on an account.	LinkedIn

(continued)

TABLE 1-2. SOCIAL MEDIA TERMS DEMYSTIFIED (CONTINUED)

TERM	DEFINITION	PLATFORM
Emoji	Small graphics that are used instead of words to convey facial expressions, actions, activities, or representations of objects.	Facebook Instagram Text Twitter
Engagement	Any type of interaction with a social media post from other accounts. These could be likes, comments, retweets, or clicks on links. Engagement is a measure of the impact of a post.	Facebook Instagram LinkedIn Twitter YouTube
Feed	A feed is an updated list of all the new content posted by the accounts a user follows on social media. Rather than being purely chronological, most social media feeds are controlled by an algorithm. Other terms used for a feed is homepage or wall.	Facebook Instagram LinkedIn Twitter
Filter	In this context, filters are used to change the appearance of an image by altering the shades, colors, or pixels in some way as an enhancement. Filters can also be used to change brightness or contrast as well as add a variety of special effects, textures, or tones to an image.	Facebook Instagram
Followers	Connections made between people and organizations by clicking the "follow" button on an account.	Instagram Twitter
Friends/fans	Connections made between people and organizations by clicking the "friend" or the "fan" button on the account.	Facebook
GIF	Animated images that are used to convey a response or feeling, without using words. Stands for "Graphics Interchange Format."	Facebook Text Twitter
Handle (@)	Think of handles as nouns. They designate and attribute a post to a particular person or an organization; any individual social media account.	Facebook Instagram LinkedIn Twitter
Hashtag (#)	Think of hashtags as descriptive. A hashtag can be a topic, an idea, or social movement; it is any word (or combination of words without spaces in between) that a community might form around. They are a tool used to aggregate posts with the hashtag, increasing its visibility to a wider audience on social media. Hashtags are searchable in the search bar of all platforms; they help people find posts that interest them and help people connect with a specific community of interest.	Facebook Instagram LinkedIn Twitter
Header image	The large photo banner that appears at the top of a social media profile.	Facebook LinkedIn Twitter YouTube

(continued)

TABLE 1-2. SOCIAL MEDIA TERMS DEMYSTIFIED (CONTINUED)

TERM	DEFINITION	PLATFORM
Home	An individual's main starting page that includes the feed (see "Feed") and links to settings that help manage and edit an account.	Facebook Twitter
Impressions	The number of times an individual's post/content is visible on another person's feed.	Facebook Instagram LinkedIn Twitter YouTube
Influencer	A social media user with a significant audience who can drive awareness about a trend, topic, company, or product.	Facebook Instagram LinkedIn Twitter YouTube
Influencer marketing	A strategy involving collaboration with an influential person on social media (an "influencer" or "micro-influencer") to promote a product, service, or campaign.	Facebook Instagram Twitter YouTube
Like	Showing support for someone else's post. It is a way to give engagement without contributing to the conversation with a comment.	Facebook Instagram LinkedIn Twitter YouTube
Mention	Tagging another social media account in a post by using the @ symbol and the account name. A notification will be sent to the recipient of the mention. Tagging is used to get the attention or give credit to other accounts in a post.	Facebook Instagram LinkedIn Twitter
Notifications	Prompts that show users when they have new followers, likes, comments, or mentions.	Facebook Instagram LinkedIn Twitter YouTube
Op-Ed: Opposite the editorial page/opinion piece	Opinion pieces that are written by persons with personalized knowledge and experience on topics of interest to the public. Usually, the pieces are 600 to 800 words and include an argument that is backed up with studies and facts.	Blog News website Newsprint
Platform	The various social media technologies that allow users to exchange digital content broadly.	Facebook Instagram LinkedIn Twitter YouTube

(continued)

TABLE 1-2. SOCIAL MEDIA TERMS DEMYSTIFIED (CONTINUED)

TERM	DEFINITION	PLATFORM
Post	Words, images, and/or video that you write and share with others in a social media platform or blog.	Facebook Instagram LinkedIn Twitter YouTube
Profile	The unique page on a social media platform that includes a person or organization's name, photos, and bio.	Facebook Instagram LinkedIn Twitter
Reply	A written response to a comment.	Facebook Instagram LinkedIn Text Twitter YouTube
Repost	An app that allows an individual to share another person's post on their own grid, giving credit to the original post.	Instagram
Retweet	When an individual shares someone else's tweet on their own Twitter profile page. This allows their followers to see the original tweet, and gives credit to the original post.	Twitter
Retweet with comment (quote retweet)	When an individual shares someone else's tweet on their own Twitter profile page, and adds a personal comment on it. This allows their followers to see the original tweet plus the comment, and gives credit to the original post.	Twitter
Share	When an individual shares someone else's post to their own wall for their followers to see.	Facebook
Tag	Adding another person's handle to your post (see "Handle" and "Mention").	Facebook Instagram LinkedIn Twitter
Timeline	A list of all of an individual's activities in chronological order.	Facebook
Tweet	A tweet is a microblog (character-limited) post on Twitter.	Twitter
Viral	A word to describe massive sharing of online content from person to person, usually in a relatively short period of time.	Facebook Instagram LinkedIn Twitter YouTube
Wall	An individual's profile page.	Facebook

Adapted from Hootsuite. (n.d.). *Dictionary of social media terms.* https://blog.hootsuite.com/social-media-definitions/

Social Media Meets Scholarship

Social media has integrated its way into scholarship. The seventh edition of the *American Psychological Association* (APA) *Publication Manual* and the eleventh edition of the *American Medical Association* (AMA) *Manual of Style* have recognized the role of online media by including a section on how to cite audiovisual media, further divided into social media, webpages, and websites (AMA, 2020a; APA, 2020). Audiovisual works may have an audio-only component (e.g., music albums, single songs, podcasts, radio interviews, speech audio recordings); visual-only component (e.g., artwork, clip art or stock images, infographics, photographs, PowerPoint slides); or both (e.g., film or video, TV series, TED Talk, webinars, YouTube videos or other streaming videos, social media, webpages, websites).

Citing Social Media

Both the APA and AMA manuals provide guidance for citing Twitter profiles and tweets, retweets, retweets with comments, and how to handle posts with emojis. Guidance is also provided for Facebook posts and pages; Instagram photos, videos, and highlights; and other online forum posts.

Citing Webpages and Websites

Webpages and websites can be used if there is not another reference category that fits or if the work has no overarching publication or parent other than the website itself. Textual works are included in the Periodicals section and provide information for citing blog posts, editorials, and use the newspaper article category for op-eds (AMA, 2020a; APA, 2020).

Bibliography Software

EndNote and other bibliography reference software programs now include templates for each of these categories to comply with the APA and AMA manuals. You will need to tweak the Output Style to match the requirements of either manual to have these references show up correctly both as in-text (narrative or parenthetical) and in the final References list.

Modern Metrics

Using social media to disseminate research is a new factor in gauging popularity and use of scholarly work. Alternative metrics factor in nontraditional citation statistics, such as the number of times a publication is tweeted or shared on social media, and are now being measured with number of traditional bibliometrics (Trueger et al., 2020).

MAKING THE CASE FOR USING SOCIAL MEDIA

Social media allows us to articulate the meaning of our work and research beyond the walls of academic journals and institutions, or in-person conversations with family and friends—it can be anywhere and anytime. It allows us to connect with patient communities and to share our health knowledge.

In our own social media journeys, we have encountered two ideas around social media use: those who use social media and those who are leery of it. Maybe you've picked up this book to take your social media game to the next level professionally. We will help you do that. Maybe you are conflicted about getting started and need more information to make your decision.

Common Objections

- You don't have time. Perhaps you are thinking that you cannot fit anything into your already busy schedule. You cannot envision how to add one more thing.
- You're not good with technology. The learning curve is too steep.
- You have imposter syndrome. You don't recognize the value of your knowledge and experience to inform others.
- It's intimidating. What will other people think of what you have to say?

Consider This

- We recommend starting with only 10 minutes per day, which can be before you start your workday, or as you finish your workday; it can be while in line at the grocery store, or during your commute on public transportation.
- Learning is good for your brain and essential for healthy aging.
- You are an expert based on your education and experience.
- You have the power to inform people with your specialized knowledge.

The conversations on social media are going on, with or without your voice. We want to help you engage and use strategies to amplify your contribution to these conversations.

SOCIAL MEDIA FOR ADVOCACY

Revolutions have been started and real change has occurred because of the explosion of social media. Social media has been called the "great equalizer." Anyone can have a Twitter or Instagram account or Facebook Page. No longer is communicating to and with the public only the job of the privileged few or those who have powerful positions or run the editorial pages of top news outlets.

For Health Care Professionals

Social media has been used to advocate for frontline workers and increase public knowledge of what nurses, physicians, respiratory therapists, and other health care professionals do, and what they need. Everyone can have a voice and those voices amplify other voices (#hcsm [health care social media]), and that is the benefit of social media. Connecting with others without a filter has never been easier.

#ShowMeYourStethoscope

You may recall an incident on *The View* in 2015 when host Joy Behar questioned why a nurse in the Miss America contest (Miss Colorado, Kelley Johnson) was "wearing a doctor's stethoscope" because apparently, nurses don't wear stethoscopes (Daley, 2015; Yahr, 2015). Nurses around the world were angry, and they shared their thoughts via social media. Behar heard from nurses through Facebook and Twitter, and she apologized after thousands of nurses posted images of themselves using the hashtag #ShowMeYourStethoscope (Daley, 2015). #ShowMeYourStethoscope carries on by becoming a "handle" @SMYSOfficial with 2900 followers and now has a Facebook Page with more than 60,000 followers as of this writing.

#IAmYourDoctor

Many physicians face frequent inappropriate comments from patients who mistake them for something other than a physician. "Where is my doctor?" or "YOU can't be a doctor?" are phrases that some physicians have to address for being too young, too black/brown, too female, too gay, too sexy, or too "different." The #IamYourDoctor social media campaign started in December 2018 on Instagram to address this discrimination, where physicians shared personal stories with each other and gave advice for how to positively respond to these types of interactions. The hashtag is still widely used to address a lack of diversity in medicine across the health care professions and to change stereotypes about what a physician should look like (Brusie, 2018).

For Public Health

While these examples may seem like a long time ago, today's COVID-19 pandemic has made the world more aware of virtual communication. During 2020, connecting with others and consuming and sharing information on social media became much more prevalent.

#COVID19

We started writing this book during the COVID-19 pandemic when health care workers were getting sick and thousands of people died because they did not have enough personal protective equipment (#PPE), intensive care unit beds, ventilators, and clinicians to run them. People were using social media to encourage

#washyourhands and stay-at-home or shelter-in-place orders; they were sharing tips on cleaning; sharing the latest evidence about the signs and symptoms of COVID-19; the numbers of confirmed cases and deaths; local, state, and federal government responses and guidelines; changes in rules and regulations regarding telehealth/telemedicine; access to care; the psychological trauma of patients dying alone; and effects the pandemic had on the world.

All of this has become more visible to the public, at least in part, because of health care professionals using social media (#MedTwitter, #Pharma, #NursesWhoTweet, #EpiTwitter) to raise awareness of workforce health issues (#NursesNeedPPE, #RTsNeedPPE).

#StopTheSpread, #WearAMask

Across all health care professions, hashtags were created on Twitter and Instagram related to preventing and slowing the spread of COVID-19. Two hashtags of #StopTheSpread and #WearAMask were eventually adopted by national organizations to further promote and advertise these public health messages (American Hospital Association, n.d.; Centers for Disease Control and Prevention, 2021).

- CDC: #StopTheSpread
- AHA: #WearAMask

#MaskUp

This hashtag started swirling around social media at the beginning of the pandemic by individuals posting selfies, or "maskies." In November 2020, thousands of hospitals around the nation banded together to create a public service message about why it was important to #MaskUp. Because of power in numbers, this campaign was able to secure full page ads in *The New York Times, USA Today, The Wall Street Journal, The Washington Post,* and *The Los Angeles Times,* and advertise on broadcast television and radio across the country (Cleveland Clinic, 2020). The American Medical Association also joined the campaign by creating a comprehensive website complete with social media assets (e.g., videos, images, graphics) asking their members to "use our campaign toolkit to share these images on social media, in your office, and anywhere in between" (AMA, 2020b).

For Social Movements

Many social movements and grassroots advocacy campaigns were started using social media, several of which were about social justice issues such as racism and oppression. The list is not exhaustive, but here are a few examples.

#BlackLivesMatter

Amplified the movement against the disproportionate murder of Black citizens by law enforcement officers.

#MeToo

Enlightened the world about the widespread sexual assault and verbal abuse on women in the workplace.

#BringBackOurGirls

The response to 276 teenage girls abducted from their boarding school in Nigeria in 2014.

For Reporting News

In today's world, the major news outlets may or may not be covering issues important to you. Social media can provide access to this information. Posts shared on social media often include macro-level word-of-mouth news about local fires, closed roads, or information about your neighborhood, schools, and kids' sports teams.

For Information

Depending on the platform, social media also provides an outlet for sharing tips for dealing with all types of stressors—from surviving the stay-at-home guidelines, homeschooling children, and dealing with financial issues because of a recently laid off spouse or partner to strategies for small businesses, health care organizations, and institutions for higher education.

Past

The way we use media to communicate has changed over time (Figure 1-1). Although we still use many of the more traditional formats, we have evolved from primarily using newspapers and radios, to digital content using computers, to mobile content using tablets and smartphones. All of us are comfortable with traditional communication methods like newsletters, email, media announcements, and phone calls; but these messages are now being amplified by social media.

Present

The COVID-19 pandemic catapulted businesses and organizations who were not on social media to use digital communication to inform local citizens about being open/closed, and how services had been adapted to meet local, state, and federal COVID safety guidelines. Social media allowed for timely information to be shared more rapidly than traditional media outlets would have allowed. Prior to COVID, examples of using social media included communication regarding the outcome of local school board meetings, school cancellations or delays due to weather, athletic event calendars, concert announcements, fundraisers, new product advertisements, and annual sales.

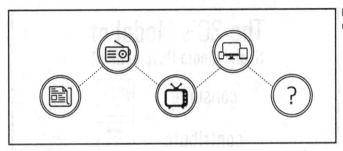

Figure 1-1. Evolution of mass communication.

Future

Post-COVID, most businesses and organizations are much more comfortable using social media because dealing with the pandemic forced them to adapt.

YOUR PROFESSIONAL EVOLUTION USING SOCIAL MEDIA

Whether you are a social media novice or have an established digital presence, our goal is to share ways that you can expand your influence and impact as a health care professional. Whether just starting out or wanting to take the next steps to up your game, we have developed the 3C's Model of Social Media Development to help guide you from the novice to expert stages: Consume -> Contribute -> Create (Figure 1-2). Each chapter breaks down the skills you need to develop or helps you see how to move to the next stage. Having a clear vision of your social media future and developing a personalized plan can guide you through the process and reduce anxiety about getting started.

Be Patient

One thing is for sure: you're not going to be an expert on day one. So relax and enjoy the process of evolving your social media skills over time. This is a marathon, not a sprint.

Expect to Zigzag

It's also not linear; this is a developmental process already happening around you, outside of you, with or without you. If you do not engage in and with social media, the public is missing out on your knowledge, experience, and perceptions of the world.

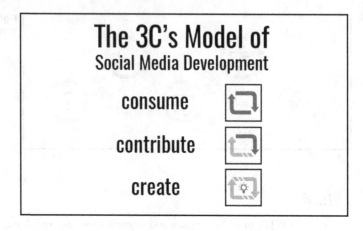

Start Slow, But Start

We believe that sharing what we know and using social media to do it is an important part of any professional practice. In today's world where information can be shared without much accountability for being credible, our expertise in health care is needed now more than ever.

NAVIGATING THE PATH TO INFLUENCE

Watch, Then Do

Think of engaging in social media the same as attending a high school dance. You wouldn't walk into the high school dance and jump right on the dance floor without knowing some of the culture and norms of such an action. That could prove to be embarrassing. You also don't need to avoid the dance floor all night—and this should be a fun and invigorating experience! Normally, you would go to the dance (get on social media) and you would begin to watch what's happening. Who's on the dance floor? Who's not? What dances are people doing? How are people acting?

```
consume ⟲
```

Cultivate Your Professional Brand

Before you go to the dance, you must know the customary attire. This is the equivalent of cultivating your professional brand—what's your look? Style? If you're like most people, your style changes over time and adapts to modern trends. Developing solid novice social media skills sets the stage for continued professional development, even if, or more likely when, the social media platforms change.

Navigating the Social Media Maze

After developing your brand, the next step on your journey is to learn about the different platforms and the ways they are designed to foster different types of content and relationships, so you know what group to join (meaning knowing what types of content are best for Facebook and how this is similar or different from content people share on Twitter, Instagram, or LinkedIn). For example, you don't want to perform a social media breakdance in a ballroom platform.

Using the Fast Lane to Build a Network

In thinking about your area of expertise and what messages you want to share, you begin to watch how others on the dance floor are behaving and the style and flow of the platform. In each of the social media platforms that you use, start by following people and organizations that interest you. Read and/or watch (Consume) what's being shared and how on various social media platforms. Start to follow targeted people and organizations.

Noise Makers and Noise Breakers

Pay attention to how specific titles catch your attention, make you want to read more, and engage with the content. These new writing skills become increasingly important as you evolve in your social media development—when you become a creator of content. Just like headlines from our favorite news sources catch our attention and keep us wanting more, observing how others craft strategic messages will become essential to building your following and creating your own content as you advance to the Contribute and Create stages.

Make Your Plan, Work Your Plan

Decide on your social media platform(s) of choice based on your target audience and main message(s). In the Consume stage, your first goals may be as simple as signing up for a particular platform for the first time, creating a profile, adding an image or logo, and learning the basics about the platform. We will guide you through how to Create a professional development plan to help you advance to the next stages.

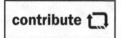

Stay Out of Hot Water

At this point, you are on social media, are watching others, and now it's time to step on the dance floor—it's time to Contribute to the conversation. At this stage of your development, you need to know the rules of the dance and how to stay out of hot water. But this is where things get more fun. You begin to add to your professional network in a virtual way, which creates a fast lane for connecting with leaders in your field. You begin to learn how to leverage the power of social media to accelerate the process of building your professional network to reach goals that are important to your career or business.

Traditional Versus Innovative Dissemination

In your current professional work, you are likely already creating traditional dissemination products such as publications and presentations. Publication in peer-reviewed scientific and clinical journals is still considered the "gold standard" for advancing science and clinical practice (and academic careers), but this historically results in a 17-year delay before 14% of original research is translated into practice and impacts patient care (Colditz & Emmons, 2018). At the Create level of social media development, you will begin to blend traditional dissemination strategies with modern social media dissemination strategies for a much more rapid translation of your work for the public, to inform practice, and to Create products for policy makers. As health care professionals our purpose is to help others and using social media to Consume, Contribute, and Create content in a fast and effective way to expand your reach. We'll also discuss how to leverage current events to elevate your voice.

Use Social Media to Connect With Traditional Media

These skills and strategies will help you build global professional relationships. Most journalists search Twitter for story ideas; 24% of verified Twitter accounts belong to journalists and news media. Cultivating your expertise online establishes trust with traditional media locally, nationally, and internationally. At this level, you can expand your influence by learning how to find and connect with journalists, and how to increase your chances of becoming an expert story source, which is good for you and your organization.

Make Your Plan, Work Your Plan

As you enter the Create stage, you are ready to initiate and lead the conga line at the high school dance. You are ready to post original content in ways that engage your audience and allows you to interact with them.

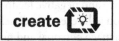

Original Content

Once you are comfortable with contributing to social via sharing content, you can then Create your own original content that others will then share. You'll learn how to adopt a new tone and writing style to make your knowledge accessible and interesting to the general public.

Thought Leadership

You will learn how to leverage current events to elevate your voice and to think about how your personal brand should guide your messages. You should consider that most everything you write should resonate with your audience and align with your public thought leadership goals, which we will help you develop. You will Create content that leaves a positive and memorable impression. Most importantly, you will provide something valuable to your followers.

Leverage Social Media

Additionally, the content that you Create on Twitter, and the skills that you will develop, will also help you to craft your own blogs and op-eds. You can use social media to share and amplify trusted sources of health care information (e.g., new evidence-based practice guidelines). You are now a person who advocates for change using social media and are an influencer and public thought leader.

Measuring Impact

As you Create content on social media, you will seek out ways to measure the impact of your social media engagement. As an individual you will learn about how you can showcase this information for your day job's annual evaluation, for promotion and tenure dossiers, and for award nominations. As a business leader you can use these metrics to develop and grow your customer base and gain insights on how your organization can improve its reach and engagement.

Managing Mistakes, Haters, and Trolls

When you reach the Create stage, you have to expect that there will be more opportunities to make mistakes; but don't let this stop you. You should certainly avoid legal and ethical pitfalls, which you can do by following the professional and organizational guidelines on social media use. Minor mistakes happen—you might have a typo in a tweet, or you might post an opinion to which others disagree. You will also realize that your content may touch some raw nerves, and that the "haters" and "trolls" might, or more likely will, challenge you. Again, this should not stop you because you also will get positive feedback—your information is useful and will resonate with others; it will provide value. But you do need to be prepared for both positive and negative feedback. The more you are in the public, the greater the chance that you will receive feedback in some form or another. We will help you to prepare for and manage personal and negative attacks that can sometimes happen.

Make Your Plan, Work Your Plan

Once you get to the Create stage, you have showcased your digital brand that is aligned with your goals, but you are not done. You can still improve and learn. While you will move back and forth between these three stages to become an ultimate influencer, you need to Create your own original content on a consistent basis. Like the dance analogy, you can improve on your dance steps and learn new ones. We will help you to Create a roadmap for planning content. You take center stage when you develop the skills to organize and plan for your own social media campaigns and capture the metrics to measure and celebrate your milestones along the way.

Your Story Has to Start Somewhere

Just like taking the dance floor, starting out on social media can be intimidating. Thoughts may run through your mind like "What if I say something stupid?" or "What if someone doesn't like my post?" We've all felt this and the best way to overcome the intimidation factor is to simply get started. The way each of us started using social media and our own evolution is different, and your story will be unique too.

Whether you decide to stay at the Consume or Contribute level—or advance to Create—this book supports all stages of development and engagement.

References

American Hospital Association. (n.d.). *Wear a mask campaign*. American Hospital Association. https://bit.ly/3q6a3UD

American Medical Association. (2020a). *AMA Manual of Style: A Guide for Authors and Editors* (11th ed.). Oxford University Press. https://doi.org/10.1093/jama/9780190246556.001.0001

American Medical Association. (2020b). *Mask Up: Stop the spread of COVID-19*. American Medical Association. https://bit.ly/350ImhN

American Psychological Association. (2020). *Publication manual of the American Psychological Association* (7th ed.). https://doi.org/https://doi.org/10.1037/0000165-000

Brown, D. (2019, December 19). *Remember Vine? These social networking sites defined the past decade*. USA Today. https://bit.ly/33hxZf2

Brusie, C. (2018, December 19). *Hashtag #IAmYourDoctor goes viral - Exposes stereotypes in healthcare*. Nurse.org. https://bit.ly/3nyVcjU

Centers for Disease Control and Prevention. (2021). *Stop the spread*. Office of the Associate Director for Communication. https://www.cdc.gov/coronavirus/2019-ncov/communication/stop-the-spread.html

Cleveland Clinic. (2020, November 19). *Thousands of top US hospitals encourage everyone to #MaskUp.* Cleveland Clinic. https://cle.clinic/3nzQPoG

Colditz, G. A., & Emmons, K. M. (2018). The promise and challenges of dissemination and implementation research. In R. C. Brownson, G. A. Colditz, & E. K. Proctor (Eds.), *Dissemination and implementation research in health: Translating science into practice* (2nd ed.). Oxford University Press.

Conten, M., Ivory , D., Yourish, K., Lai, R., Hassan, A., Calderone, J., Smith, M., Lemonides, A., Allen, J., Blair, S., Burakoff, M., Cahalan, S., Cassel, Z., Craig, M., De Jesus, Y., Dupré, B., Facciola, T., Fortis, B., Gorenflo, G., Higgins, L., Holland, J., ... (2020, August 13). *About 38% of U.S. coronavirus deaths are linked to nursing homes.* The New York Times. https://nyti.ms/31mkr1B

Gayton C. (2020, July 18). *The origins of TikTok.* ChristinaGayton.medium.com. https://bit.ly/3uNlFxJ

Gil, R. (2019, December 19). *The evolution of social media advertising.* IAS insider. https://bit.ly/30qLVvw

Hendricks, D. (2019, November 2, 2020). *Complete history of social media: Then and now.* Small Business Trends. https://bit.ly/3cENGQD

Hootsuite. (n.d.). *Dictionary of social media terms.* https://blog.hootsuite.com/social-media-definitions/

Kemp, S. (2020, November 2). *Digital 2020: Global digital overview.* Datareportal. https://bit.ly/3jNMMn2

McFadden, C. (2020, November 2). *A chronological history of social media.* Interesting Engineering. https://bit.ly/2GfC5eE

Merriam-Webster. (2020, November 4). Social media. Merriam-Webster.com dictionary. https://bit.ly/2TZfVAV

Nguyen T. (2021, February 10). *Clubhouse, the invite-only audio app, explained.* Vox.com. https://bit.ly/3fOho9f

O'Connell B. (2020, February 28). *History of snapchat: Timeline and facts.* TheStreet.com. https://bit.ly/3yUbrPD

Oxford English Dictionary. (November 4, 2020). Tweet. Oxford English Dictionary. https://www.oed.com

Samur, A. (2018, November 22). *The history of social media: 29+ key moments.* Hootsuite. https://bit.ly/3856kBa

Schumacher, S., & Kent, N. (2020, April 2). *8 charts on internet use around the world as countries grapple with COVID-19.* Pew Research Center. https://pewrsch.ch/34N1UfW

Shearer, E., & Grieco, E. (2019, October 2). *Americans are wary of the role social media sites play in delivering the news.* Pew Research Center. https://pewrsr.ch/2TOdZeJ

Trueger, N., Yilmaz, Y., & Chan, T. (2020). Leveraging tweets, citations, and social networks to improve bibliometrics. *JAMA Network Open,* 3(7), e2010911. https://doi.org/10.1001/jamanetworkopen.2020.10911

Van Dijck, J. (2013). *The culture of connectivity: A critical history of social media.* Oxford University Press.

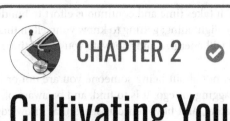

CHAPTER 2

Cultivating Your Professional Brand

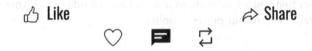

👍 Like   ↪ Share

♡   🗨   ⇄

> "There is power in allowing yourself to be known and heard, in owning your unique story, in using your authentic voice."
>
> *Michelle Obama*
> *@MichelleObama*

Know thyself. Everyone has a brand—whether by design or default. Sometimes life moves too fast for us to stop and think about this. But it's important as a professional and as a human with a digital footprint to consider how to make the most of this for yourself and your professional goals.

With social media, you are representing yourself with every post you share. If you don't take the time to develop your brand, who you think you are might not necessarily be how you are perceived. Self-awareness is a major component in this process and getting feedback from trusted colleagues can help verify your findings during the branding process.

KEEP IT FUN, BUT REAL

The branding process is an opportunity to reflect on your unique personality, what is important to you, the expertise you have to share, and what your goals are for expanding your audience and influence. This doesn't happen overnight. While

Shattell, M., Batchelor, M., & Darmoc, R. *Social Media in Health Care:
A Guide to Creating Your Professional Digital Presence* (pp. 25-38).
© 2022 Taylor & Francis Group.

this chapter will help you get started, it takes time and continuous effort to build your brand. But we can promise it will be enlightening; getting to know yourself in this new way and seeing how people respond will energize and motivate you to continue your journey to social influence.

The goal of personal branding is not about being someone you are not or being fake. It is not about exaggerating, bragging, or ego. It is to find, and be aware of, your personal and professional differentiators, and how you can share that knowledge in your own way.

Becoming a social influencer in health care is about providing value. What unique value can you offer your desired audience? This chapter will help you define your personal brand as an expert—who you are and who your audience is so you can stay focused on delivering valuable content that will resonate with their needs.

Remember that you are defining your authentic, real-life brand. Then we will show you how to transfer it to your presence online.

WHAT MAKES A BRAND?

We usually think of brands as names, products, logos, or taglines, but these are just elements of the brand. The true essence of a brand is all the word associations or key words left over in people's minds after they have an encounter or experience with you—whether in person or online.

Think of your brand as a promise to your audience to deliver something trustworthy and reliable. It's more than just the product being sold. It's the unique value proposition that differentiates one brand (your brand) from all others. To understand how to develop your brand, let's look at some successful examples from corporate and celebrity brands.

Learning From Corporate Brands

All corporate brands that sell products have functional benefits—quality, cost, taste, smell, or reliability depending on the type of product. But the best, and largest, brands know that functional benefits are not enough to win the hearts and minds of loyal customers. Brands must develop higher-level emotional connections with their core audience. This serves to not only make each customer feel a connection to the brand that matches their higher level emotional needs, but also makes them want to align themselves with the brand. When a consumer buys a t-shirt, cup, or hat displaying the brand logo, this signifies to the world that they identify with the brand's personality and values.

Branding #Coffee

Who doesn't love, or need, coffee? Will you drink just any type of coffee? When you think of big coffee brands like Starbucks or Nespresso or Dunkin' (Donuts), do you have a different inherent feeling about each of these? You should, because it was designed that way. Branding coffee is more than just about the functional benefits of taste, cost, and variety of products. Each of these three brands have a different identity, personality, and target audience. They follow through on their brand promise in the way you experience the product.

@Starbucks

Starbucks brand is urban, modern, friendly, high quality, consistent, ethical, cool. Starbucks popularized the term "baristas" to refer to their employees, elevating them from cashiers and people who pour ingredients into your cup, to coffee-making specialists. Their stores are known for welcoming patrons to stay for a while; many people bring their laptop and work, meet up with friends, or catch up with neighbors for a chat while enjoying their beverage and gourmet snack. Starbucks also cares about sustainability—ethical sourcing of ingredients, supporting farmers, and taking it a step further most recently in 2020, committing to cut greenhouse gas emissions, eliminating waste, and conserving water by 50% over the next 10 years (Warnick, 2020).

@Nespresso

Nespresso's brand is exclusive, sophisticated, innovative, luxurious, has international relationships, and is grounded in community (Nespresso, 2020). Nespresso arguably offers the most beautiful at-home machines to brew their attractive metallic espresso pods. Consumers with expensive taste gravitate toward their personality of luxury, with George Clooney as spokesperson in their advertising and a community for the Nespresso Club. The brand promotes European flavors and rare coffees from all over the world, while also stressing the importance of their relationships with farmers, protecting the environment, and recycling. Nespresso fans resonate with their line of "Reviving Origins" coffee and stories told about the far-away lands where each originates.

@Dunkin'

Dunkin's brand is fast, fun, convenient, affordable, bold, youthful, iconic (Dunkin' Donuts, 2018). Rebranded from Dunkin' Donuts to just Dunkin' in 2019, the brand kept their retro colors of pink and orange and modernized the other graphics for a more youthful look, but kept the throwback feeling of the iconic Dunkin' Donuts brand and the heritage that is still relevant and memorable to today's customers. Sometimes companies create their own slogans and sometimes a customer will go viral with an expression of their own to inadvertently promote the brand, as was the case with a woman from Boston who was voting in the 2020 Presidential election. A television news crew was interviewing people in line at Fenway Park, and in her short interview the woman commented animatedly in a Boston accent "I got my Dunkie's!" and held up her branded Dunkin' cup. The video went viral because it was "so Boston" and was viewed on Twitter 1.7 million times that day (Puhak, 2020). #GotMyDunkies is a fun and youthful slogan that matches the brand personality of Dunkin' and was priceless publicity.

All of these coffee brands are highly successful and memorable because they have positioned themselves with emotional and functional associations in the minds of customers, which the brand follows through on in every interaction. So, it's not just about the coffee. Each brand is a promise of what customers will get: what they will feel, how the brand will deliver it, and the collection of all the expectations people carry about them. This corporate example was about coffee, but it shows how unique branding and marketing make each of them distinct from each other, appealing to different audiences.

People as Brands

Today when we talk about brands, we're no longer just talking about companies. We're talking about people. Politicians, actors, musicians, and athletes all have their own brand. And, like their corporate counterparts, they too face the challenge of remaining relevant to their audience.

Current celebrities with strong brands are Taylor Swift, the Kardashians, LeBron James, Martha Stewart, Tiger Woods, and Beyoncé. You may or may not like them, but the power of their brands are recognizable and undeniable.

Dr. Anthony Fauci

As an employee of the National Institute of Allergy and Infectious Diseases (@NIAIDNews), Dr. Anthony Fauci is a physician and immunologist; a world expert on infectious disease. He was named one of the most trusted medical figures in the United States, most cited scientist across all scientific journals, and presented with the Presidential Medal of Freedom. During the COVID-19 pandemic, he led the White House Coronavirus Task Force and was the source of truth for most of America because of his credibility and experience. But the first year of the pandemic was politically charged, with conflicting misinformation both in traditional and social media from people in power. Fauci had to defend his reputation numerous times, and even made an appearance on *60 Minutes* to reinforce his brand as a trusted scientist whose singular goal was to protect the American public from the novel disease.

Celebrity Doctors

Let's look at two health care professionals who earned celebrity status and how their brand has changed over time as their popularity and influence increased.

@DrOz

Dr. Mehmet Oz went from cardiothoracic surgeon to health educator and sometimes pseudoscience promoter. He gained popularity from national morning news appearances, books, and eventually his own television show. His topics centered mainly around food, healthy eating, and every fad diet that ever existed, but also topics that were in no way related to his specialty, or health care at all. Criticized by other physicians for promoting alternative medicine and unscientific findings for a wide range of issues, *The Dr. Oz Show* went with the demands of an audience looking for new and not necessarily scientific information, while still claiming his brand and respect as a physician.

@DrPhil

Dr. Phil McGraw went from clinical psychologist and life coach to pop culture therapist on sensational topics (brand/audience went from Oprah to Jerry Springer). He made more than 60 appearances on *The Oprah Winfrey Show* to promote his books, and because of his success was offered his own television show. Although his tough love advice remained the same for *Dr. Phil*, it is clear to see his brand transformation in the following television show topics while he was on *The Oprah Winfrey Show* compared to when he had his own talk show.

Dr. Phil on *Oprah* show topics (life coaching):

- Getting past your fear of failure
- Making peace with your parents
- How to move on after a break-up

Dr. Phil show topics (sensational):

- My sister is a total train wreck
- My teen is a wild child
- Too much drama!
- He's a cheater: the polygraph results

We would have to ask Drs. Oz and Phil why their brands changed. It is clear there was a change in audience, with most likely a change of purpose or motivation. Maybe they wanted to build their own empire with a larger audience or focus on what sells on daytime TV to get more money from corporate advertising.

These are extreme examples of success. Without judgment on their personal branding decisions, we can see how health care professionals branded, or rebranded, themselves based on their audience and goals.

BUILDING TRUST FOR YOUR PROFESSIONAL BRAND

We talked about corporate brands, but did you know that only 37% of people in the United States trust corporate communications from brands they use or buy? (Edelman, 2019, 2020). Inversely, study after study shows that individuals earn more trust and influence than brands. On social media, 61% of people find "a person like me" to be credible or very credible. This indicates that real people can have more influence than celebrities or corporate brands.

Why Is This?

Because as much as people might love a particular brand, they know these companies are ultimately driven by profit. We see their messages as advertisements. And of course, a corporate brand is never going to say anything bad about their brand or product. Corporate brands are, consciously or unconsciously, viewed as machines backed by public relations departments, crisis communications experts, and highly paid financial executives in the C-suite. This shift in trust and media consumption offers an opportunity for health care professionals.

BUILDING INDIVIDUAL TRUST

The Trust Barometer study had another crucial finding: the only two groups of people who are trusted more than "people like me" and rated "very or extremely credible" are academic experts and company technical experts—for health care, this means clinicians or executives. If you are a health care professional or an academic—or both—your education and training establish a large part of your authority. You have the power to influence others because of your status as a professor, clinician, or health advocate. You have already earned the respect of the public through your involvement in higher education and experts at your health care organization. Here are some easy ways to Contribute in your journey to start building influence.

Word of Mouth

In today's world, most consumers will ask friends for recommendations and reviews of personal experience before making decisions (e.g., asking your friends online for their recommendations on where to stay, where to eat, or personal experience with certain products). Word of mouth has always been a gold standard way to determine what you could or should do in each situation, and social media allows for rapid responses from your circle of friends and acquaintances, and even from the general public. More often, we look for and read reviews from real people before making any decision (not paid advertisers or corporations).

Online Reviews

How many times have you looked up information about the best hotels, or restaurants, or pair of shoes? Which do you trust more—what the company says on its website, or the reviews people have written about them? Websites are great for getting a feel for the brand experience, but customer feedback gives you more insight into what is real and what is fluff from the corporate brand communications. Online reviews and recommendations are even the norm for hospitals, health systems, individual health care professionals, and universities.

Now it's time for you to decide how you want to use your individual respect, trust, and authority.

You—The Brand

Imagine for a moment that you are also a brand. You set expectations. You make promises. You deliver expert communications, and you are evaluated based on your perceived brand.

The goal is to start the process of helping you develop a well-thought-out, strong, confident, authentic personal brand where you help others, have a positive impact, and achieve your personal and professional goals.

By Design

For online influence you have to intentionally develop your brand, and you don't have to be famous to do this. As mentioned earlier, everyone has a brand; it's up to you to articulate and solidify it with your presence and actions online. The personal branding process is a fun, easy, and painless way to get up to date on who you are and what you do. It shines a spotlight on your talents and clearly identifies your impact on the people you interact with.

The Process

Building Personality

To begin this process, you should write down a list of key words that encapsulate who you are, and what you want people to remember about you. If you can't think of words right away, use the list in Table 2-1 as a guide and pick 10 words that resonate the most with you and your professional presence (Lead Through Strengths, n.d.).

Your word selections should be authentic. Ask a trusted colleague or friend to see if what you think about yourself is what you actually put out into the world. Tell them you are doing some branding work and ask for candid feedback on whether your key words resonate. If not, don't get rid of your words if you feel strongly about them. This is a great opportunity to intentionally focus on who you are, and pivot to amplify your desired brand during interactions with others. Always aspire for what you want to be.

TABLE 2-1. PERSONALITY ADJECTIVES FOR PROFESSIONAL BRANDING

Accessible	Confident	Effortless	Groundbreaking
Accommodating	Confrontational	Elaborate	Growth focused
Accountable	Consistent	Elegant	Happy
Action-oriented	Conscientious	Empathetic	Hardworking
Active	Contemplative	Encouraging	Harmonious
Adaptable	Contemporary	Enduring	Healthy
Adventurous	Contrarian	Energetic	Helpful
Altruistic	Controlled	Engaging	High-touch
Ambitious	Cool	Enterprising	Holistic
Anticipating	Cooperative	Entertaining	Honest
Assertive	Conversational	Enthusiastic	Honorable
Astute	Courageous	Equitable	Hopeful
Attentive	Creative	Excellence seeking	Humble
Bold	Curious	Exclusive	Imaginative
Brave	Custom	Exploring	Impactful
Bright	Cutting edge	Extroverted	Impartial
Calm	Daring	Factual	Independent
Candid	Data-driven	Fair	Initiating
Captivating	Decisive	Faithful	Intuitive
Careful	Deep	Fascinating	Innovative
Caring	Dependable	Fearless	Inquisitive
Casual	Determined	Fierce	Insightful
Cautious	Dignified	Fixing	Inspiring
Celebrating	Diligent	Flexible	Instigating
Challenging	Diplomatic	Formal	Instinctive
Change-ready	Direct	Forward thinking	Integrative
Charismatic	Discerning	Frank	Intellectual
Charming	Disruptive	Fresh	Intense
Chic	Driven	Friendly	Intentional
Classic	Dutiful	Fun	Interactive
Clever	Dynamic	Funny	Intriguing
Collaborative	Eager	Futuristic	Intuitive
Colorful	Early adopting	Generous	Inventive
Comforting	Easygoing	Genuine	Intimate
Committed	Eccentric	Goal-oriented	Introspective
Competitive	Edgy	Gregarious	Investigating
Concentrated	Efficient	Grounded	Inviting

(continued)

TABLE 2-1. PERSONALITY ADJECTIVES FOR PROFESSIONAL BRANDING (CONTINUED)

Irreverent	Peaceful	Resolute	Systematic
Joyful	Perceptive	Resourceful	Tactful
Juggling	Persevering	Responsive	Tactical
Kind	Persistent	Revealing	Tenacious
Level	Persuasive	Righteous	Thoughtful
Lively	Philosophical	Routine	Timeless
Logical	Planned	Rugged	Tireless
Low maintenance	Playful	Safe	Tolerant
Loyal	Poetic	Scrappy	Traditional
Luxurious	Polished	Seeking	Transforming
Magnetic	Polite	Selective	Transparent
Measured	Posh	Selfless	Trendy
Methodical	Positive	Self-sufficient	Trend spotter
Meticulous	Powerful	Sensible	Troubleshooting
Mindful	Practical	Serious	Trustworthy
Modern	Pragmatic	Sharp	Unbiased
Modest	Predictable	Sincere	Unbound
Momentum creator	Present	Singular	Unconventional
Multi-passionate	Principled	Skeptical	Understanding
Musing	Private	Sleek	Unifying
Mysterious	Provocative	Sociable	Unique
Natural	Proud	Solid	Upbeat
Noble	Purposeful	Sophisticated	Urban
Noisy	Questioning	Soulful	Values-driven
Nostalgic	Quick	Spontaneous	Variety seeking
Nurturing	Quiet-spoken	Stable	Versatile
Observant	Quirky	Standard	Vibrant
Open-minded	Rational	Steadfast	Vigorous
Opinionated	Raw	Stimulating	Vivid
Optimistic	Realistic	Stoic	Warm
Orderly	Reasoned	Straightforward	Welcoming
Organized	Receptive	Strategic	Whimsical
Original	Reflective	Striking	Winning
Outgoing	Refreshing	Striving	Wise
Passionate	Relaxing	Structured	Witty
Patient	Reliable	Successful	Worldly
Pattern spotting	Resilient	Sympathetic	Zealous

TABLE 2-2. WHAT IS YOUR AREA OF EXPERTISE AND KNOWLEDGE?

CLINICAL EXPERTISE/ PROFESSIONAL BACKGROUND	AREA OF SCHOLARSHIP/ TEACHING EXPERTISE	LEADERSHIP SKILLS/ UNIQUE ACTIVITIES OR PERSPECTIVES
Family nurse practitioner	Cardiovascular health; online education	Motivational interviewing; marathon runner
Geriatric psychiatrist	Alzheimer's disease and related dementias	Creativity and art-based therapy
Child and adolescent mental health	Suicide risk behaviors; cutting; gaming/simulation	Group therapy; residential treatment; family caregiver
Hospital operations executive	Age-friendly health systems; inclusive excellence	Strategic planning; Responsibility Center Management budget models; Vice-President of American Hospital Association

Building Credibility

Now it's time to move on to your unique professional education, experience, and expertise. Use this chart to help you solidify your specialty areas, education, credentials, accolades, and unique differentiators (Table 2-2).

Building Goals

Being clear about your goals for using social media is crucial in the branding process. Your passions, ideas, and purpose all drive your ultimate goals, and will help you decide on your audience. While you may have multiple answers for the questions posed in the sample chart, it is important to write down your goals and get clear about your purpose to inform development of a well-defined brand in which your primary audience finds value (Table 2-3).

Building an Audience

At the heart of every successful brand design is identifying your primary audience. Deciding on who you want to reach will allow you to focus on the information that will be most interesting, useful, and unique to them. It is also your path to differentiation among others with the same audience. Many of you will want to have, or think you have, multiple audiences. This approach is okay if you always have your primary audience defined and kept in mind when posting content. Your primary audience will be the most loyal part of your network; they will engage with you and look to you for compelling information. Most importantly, they will remember you.

Table 2-3. Defining Your Goals and Purpose

WHAT ARE YOU PASSIONATE ABOUT?	WHAT IDEAS DO YOU HAVE TO SHARE?	WHAT IS YOUR GOAL?	WHO DO YOU WANT TO REACH?
Convincing patients that whole health is crucial.	Tips about nutrition, medication, exercise, mental health.	Help as many people as possible by sharing my ideas.	The general public and people living with heart disease or diabetes.
Fighting for access to health care for all people.	Stories from my underserved patients.	Influence policy.	The media; politicians; related non-profit organizations.
Mentoring others.	Successful ways to overcome obstacles.	Become a thought leader on "x" topic.	Industry colleagues and new "x" professionals.
Changing/ improving the system.	Innovative ways that I practice.	Move from clinician to executive/leader position.	Industry executives and organizations.
My "x" area of expertise and how it can help people/ change their lives.	Specific ways I can help "x" patients. Insights from my research.	Expand my practice and research funding. Build a legacy.	The media; organizations and colleagues in the same specialty.

Objections in the Process

We have found that some people are uncomfortable with the idea of promoting themselves or shining a spotlight on their work.

> **"Without promotion something terrible happens ... nothing!"**
> *P. T. Barnum*

Owning Your Value

Don't be afraid of self-promotion. You should proudly claim your expertise and accomplishments that you earned through education, experience, and dedication. If you are not out there promoting yourself and your important work, no one else will do it for you.

We need to reframe "self-promotion"—it is not a dirty word. You most likely pursued a career in health care to help people; promoting what you do through social media allows you to reach more people and affect more lives almost immediately.

Transitioning Your Brand to Social Media

Your brand starts with your bio. Once you develop your authentic personal brand, it's time to transition it to your online persona by crafting your bio with the most important words and phrases that demonstrate your personality, credibility, and best connect with your audience.

Elements of Your Bio

Sign up for a social account on LinkedIn and Twitter (or Instagram or Facebook if you choose), or edit your current ones while keeping these tips in mind.

Name/@Handle

Always use your real name, if possible. It makes you easier to find during an online search and activates your memorability.

Profile Photo

For credibility, you must have a profile photo. We recommend using the same photo across professional social platforms for easier recognition and branding. Seeing a person's face forms an emotional connection in our brains and allows us to create more meaningful relationships online. Make sure your profile photo is current, not one from 20 years ago, to keep your brand authentic.

Header Photo

For platforms that allow header photos like Twitter, LinkedIn, Facebook, and YouTube, find a photo of yourself in action, whether speaking at a conference, in your clinical setting, with a group of colleagues, or at your workplace. These photos will lend additional credibility to your brand and show your unique personality.

Website

The bio section of all platforms is a place to add a website URL. You can add your faculty or clinician profile from your organization's website, your LinkedIn profile URL, or your personal website (if you have one). The key is to include something where people can verify that you are who you say that you are. A reporter or organization might see one of your tweets, but if they don't have a way to confirm that you are a legitimate expert working at a well-known organization or in your own practice, they will move on to the next person.

Description

On Twitter, you only have 160 characters to describe yourself; remember your brand, to highlight what you offer. Frame yourself as an authority. Use key words that reflect your areas of expertise in your industry so people can find you. Add your place of work with its social media handle. If you are a member of a prestigious organization, add it. Key words that reflect your areas of expertise will increase search visibility for journalists and peers looking for an expert.

Disclaimer

Although free speech is guaranteed, it's imperative to separate your opinion from that of your employer. A blatantly offensive, discriminating, or vulgar post on social media is likely to cause your human resources department to take action toward you regardless of a disclaimer, and most professionals know where the line is. Be sure to write some variation of the idea that your posts reflect your opinion and not the opinion or views of your employer. With only 160 total characters on Twitter, you need to get creative. Here are a few options on how to shorten this disclaimer: "Opinions are my own and not the views of my employer"; "My tweets are my own"; "Opinions are mine"; "Views = own."

Look at the social bios of people you respect in your profession to get ideas for how to strategically form the best bio for your brand. Remember that you can change your bio at any time, so have fun with it and try out different words and phrases.

YOUR PROFESSIONAL PRESENCE IS DIGITAL

You've got your personal brand and your Twitter and/or other social media bio set up.

You have immense experience in health care that can benefit many depending on your goals and how willing you are to share it publicly with your authentic voice.

Deciding where to share and learning how each social platform works is the next step in building your digital presence.

REFERENCES

Dunkin' Donuts. (2018, September 25). *Welcome to Dunkin': Dunkin' Donuts reveals new brand identity.* Dunkin' Donuts. https://bit.ly/2Wr8V1d

Edelman. (2019, June 18). *Edelman trust barometer special report: In brands we trust?* Edelman. https://bit.ly/3nC8ahQ

Edelman. (2020, January 19). 2020 *Edelman trust barometer.* Edelman. https://bit.ly/2Wu8fIw

Lead Through Strengths. (n.d.). *List of adjectives for your personal career brand.* Lead Through Strengths. https://bit.ly/3hYp7Ri

Nespresso. (2020). *Home page.* Nespresso. https://www.nespresso.com/us/en/

Puhak, J. (2020, October 20). *Dunkin'-drinking Boston woman goes viral following interview in early-voting line: 'Got my Dunkies'.* Fox News. https://fxn.ws/3qcVI9o

Warnick, J. (2020, December 18). *5 things to know about Starbucks new environmental sustainability policy.* Starbucks Stories and News. https://bit.ly/2KbOXVM

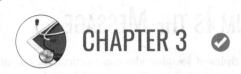

CHAPTER 3 ✅

Maneuvering the Social Media Maze

👍 Like   ↪ Share

♡   💬   🔁

"A journey of a thousand miles begins with a single step."

Lao Tzu

Maneuvering social media can be as overwhelming as being lost in a maze. Just as our stories are different for how we got started with social media, there are many ways to engage with social media. Everyone will have a different timeline. Getting started or adding to your repertoire doesn't have to feel like you are in a maze, and you don't have to be on every social media platform to make an impact. In fact, we recommend that you strategically choose one social media platform that connects you to your largest desired audience, and then add other platforms as you develop your social media skills. The purpose of this chapter is to give you a 30,000-foot overview of what's out there and how each platform can be used.

The social media landscape changes as technology evolves, so there will always be new platforms created. Currently, 4.62 billion people use social media—that's half of the world's population, with growth rates of 2 million new users per day (DataReportal, 2022). Our focus will be on platforms most often used in the health care industry. Some platforms can be blended with personal use, depending on your target audience, intention, and goal.

Shattell, M., Batchelor, M., & Darmoc, R. *Social Media in Health Care: A Guide to Creating Your Professional Digital Presence* (pp. 39-54). © 2022 Taylor & Francis Group.

The Medium Is the Message

When thinking about the principles of social media communication, one of the best minds to help us learn is Marshall McLuhan (Gordon, 2002). McLuhan didn't have the opportunity to experience social media the way we know it today, but that didn't stop him from exerting a huge influence on it. During his career, McLuhan spoke about technology and communication creating a "global village," just as social media has done to connect us with others from around the world. As an educator of communication and its evolution over time, McLuhan introduced many concepts about the impact of new media. But McLuhan's theory, "The medium is the message," has had a definitive impact on media in general, which can also be applied to social media (McLuhan, 1964).

Elements of the Theory

"The medium is the message" means that the medium (or platform) we use to communicate is as valuable as the message itself. The medium can be radio, television, print, film, the internet, and now social media. The central idea is that the medium is imperative to the way that content (the message) is perceived.

Effect of New Mediums

We can easily see how a new medium can affect us. Before the telephone, there was no such thing as having a conversation with a friend or colleague in another city or state, at least not without a long physical journey. Today, we are always just a phone call away from a friend or family member, even internationally. We have become used to communicating with each other easily. Now many of us don't even use the telephone, we Zoom on a video call or send a text to communicate. We can see this with digital and social media today; the way we get our news and information about what is happening in the world and in our communities has drastically changed. How does this new digital medium of social media affect the messages we want to communicate? Some real-life comparisons can help us understand this theory.

Game of Thrones

Even if you haven't experienced *Game of Thrones* (GOT), you most likely have heard about it. GOT started out as a book series, then a 1-hour television series with eight seasons, and even has an interactive website where users dictate the plotline that includes GOT people, places, and things. In comparing the three different mediums used to tell this story, you can see how the user experience is different. The book and the television series are both linear—you passively read or watch as the story unfolds from beginning to end in an order developed by the author and/or director. In contrast, the website allows users to be the orchestrator of the story, clicking on different links and sections to determine the history and interactions of characters and plots.

Bieber Fever

The traditional trajectory of a musician being discovered would be playing gigs at clubs and eventually being discovered by a record label. The artist's music would be heard by the public on the radio or featured on a late-night television show. Contrast this to today's world where Justin Bieber, as a young teenager, created a YouTube Channel where he posted videos of himself singing. He didn't go through the usual steps that musical artists of the past did to achieve success in the industry. YouTube, as a medium, provided him exposure to music producers and agents that was not available to previous generations.

Medium + Message

Think about how your content will use social media, as a medium and as a message. In the #BlackLivesMatter movement, Twitter became the medium of choice in every way: from finding like-minded individuals, to sharing real-life stories, to groups that organized across the nation to protest, to global news coverage. Twitter stood out because it enabled people to connect and communicate in real time—from anywhere.

The Takeaway

For social media, how do we utilize McLuhan's theory, "The medium is the message"? It starts as soon as an idea comes to us. As professionals, we need to guide our audience down the right path with the right information, located on the right platform. The way you experience video on Instagram is different than the way you experience it on YouTube or Twitter.

Staying true to the message and the medium goes hand in hand with building your brand, all of which are adaptive and constantly expanding with technology and new mediums. You must select the social platform that aligns with the content you have to share.

OVERVIEW OF SOCIAL MEDIA PLATFORMS

The principles for strategically using social media are timeless, so let's dive right into the key platforms for social influence. The major social media platforms for health care professionals are Facebook, Twitter, LinkedIn, Instagram, and YouTube. Play around with the platforms. You are not going to break anything, so explore. Click on different people, links, photos, and words so you can become familiar with how each platform works.

Facebook: 2.91 Billion Active Users (DataReportal, 2022)

Facebook is the most widely used across demographics but focuses mainly on personal connections. Being "friends" on Facebook has more of a personal rather than professional feel, although this is evolving. Facebook allows you to have a personal (private) account and a public-facing page. There are groups on Facebook that might help you if you are a researcher looking for a specific audience with which to connect (e.g., parenting groups, older adults, hobbyists). If you have your own company or business that you want to promote, you can set it up as a "page." This is not to say that you cannot post your work (articles or blog posts) or share health information, but the main purpose and audience on Facebook remains family and friends. There are other platforms that can be better for health care professionals who may want to grow their business, connect with industry leaders, or find groups for possible collaborators or research participants.

Facebook Page

Most businesses will have a Facebook Page (comparable to a profile for individuals) that you can follow to stay connected and build your professional and organizational network. As an individual, use your Facebook Page to promote your podcast, events where you will be speaking, or events you will host in your leadership role. Your Facebook Page is also the site you use to share Facebook Live content for public consumption.

Facebook Live

Looking for a better way to increase engagement? Facebook Live gives you a platform to engage and interact with your audience and record the Live sessions to use later. Streaming and recording allows you to share events with a broader audience during and after the event and use your analytics to report your impact.

Repurpose Video

The recorded videos can also be used to create microcontent to promote across platforms. Microcontent is a 30-second to 1-minute video from a larger video file. Microcontent is created using a micro/clip in iMovie that you can share across platforms with a graphic or quote to amplify the clip's key message.

Cover Events

Other ways Facebook Live can be used is to cover a poster presentation by a colleague at a conference—allowing not only conference-goers to view the poster but giving an opportunity to share with a larger, broader audience the scholarship being presented. Be sure to know the "rules" of the conference you are attending, as well as privacy concerns.

Incorporate Data Into Reports

These links can also be helpful in demonstrating outcomes (deliverables) as part of a grant to share with the funders.

Twitter: 436 Million Active Users (DataReportal, 2022)

Tweets are made in real-time, so it is more current than the news on TV or online because you can use hashtags to find news that no one is reporting on. Twitter is used by individuals and organizations to post information, to promote work, and to share knowledge with policy makers and journalists. You can post images along with text but have a maximum of 280 characters. Succinct clear writing works best in tweets (a "tweet" is a noun that represents the post, "Twitter" is the platform). We will focus on Twitter later in this chapter and in the rest of the book.

LinkedIn: 810 Million Users (LinkedIn, 2022)

Creating a LinkedIn profile is essential for credibility. Think of it as a CliffsNotes version of your résumé. It's a way to verify your identity and showcase your education, your previous and current job positions, years of experience, awards and accomplishments, and a selection of prominent publications that your audience will find most interesting. However, LinkedIn inherently has less engagement—only 1% of users share content on a weekly basis (Osman, 2020). Most members simply use it to browse for people in their organization, their industry, or use it to find out more about a new acquaintance. It is also a tool that employment recruiters use to find candidates for open positions; about 87% of recruiters use LinkedIn. While you might not choose to post on LinkedIn regularly, you do need to keep your profile updated because many times when people search your name online, this is the first place you will show up in the Google search results.

For the Pros

LinkedIn is the largest professionally focused social platform and is geared toward career development and professional networking. LinkedIn allows you to post your résumé, search for jobs or internships, learn skills to succeed in your career, and post updates that enhance your professional reputation. LinkedIn allows you to post your educational background, work experience, special skills, and make recommendations for colleagues. You can post videos and/or photos, organize offline events, and join groups that are of interest to your career.

Instagram: 1.48 Billion Active Users (DataReportal, 2022)

Now owned by Facebook, Instagram is an app developed for sharing photos and videos from a mobile device. You must use your own digital photos and videos or know how to create graphic images. The general audience is slightly different than those on Facebook and the two do work together; you can configure Instagram to post photos on Facebook, Twitter, or Tumblr. Videos up to 60 seconds in length can be posted, and there is an option to "go live" just like Facebook. Photos and videos taken with Instagram can be enhanced with more than 40 filters. Getting people to engage with your content will generate more followers. Having more followers and using hashtags means you will show up in more feeds and people will find your account. For example, if you want to build up your clinical practice, you might include patient testimonials and photos of your office and staff. You can share tips for patients based on your specialty; a cardiologist might share nutrition and exercise tips for a healthy heart, or a mental health clinician could share meditation practices or quotes about how to deal with stress. If you don't have a photo or video for this content, using design apps (e.g., Canva, WordSwag) to change text into images is necessary for posting on Instagram.

Instagram Stories

Stories allows you to link together multiple clips in a slideshow format; photo and graphic clips show up for 7 seconds while video clips can be up to 15 seconds. Once you post a clip to your story, only your followers can see it and it only stays on your account for 24 hours then disappears, unless you save it as a "highlight" on your profile. You can add text, music, stickers, and GIFs to your stories.

Instagram Reels

Reels are 30-second multiple-clip videos that can be seen by anyone if you choose. They allow for creative video editing and messaging directly on the video, with the option to add music and special effects.

YouTube: 2.56 Billion Active Users (DataReportal, 2022)

YouTube is the second largest search engine on the internet after Google (Wagner, 2017). YouTube allows you to share videos and host them in one place. If you want to do video snippets to use as content for your other social media channels, YouTube is the place to start. This platform is extremely popular for video tutorials, product reviews, pranks, comedy sketches, unboxing reveals, educational content, and watching video games. Unlike Twitter, Instagram, Facebook, or LinkedIn, YouTube videos are searchable, which gives you a distinct advantage if you are interested in growing your audience and upping your level of engagement (Cannell & Travis, 2018). For professionals, we recommend using it as a hosting platform to upload your own brand-related videos, then sharing the video links on your other social accounts.

TABLE 3-1. CHARACTER LIMITS AND IDEAL LENGTH FOR POSTS				
	MAXIMUM LENGTH OF CHARACTERS	IDEAL LENGTH OF CHARACTERS	MAXIMUM NUMBER OF HASHTAGS	IDEAL NUMBER OF HASHTAGS
FACEBOOK	63,206	40 to 80	No limit	1 to 4
TWITTER	280	71 to 100	No limit	1 to 2
LINKEDIN	1295	50 to 100	No limit	3 to 5
INSTAGRAM	2200	138 to 150	30	5 to 10
YOUTUBE	5000	150 or more	15	2 to 3

Character Counts

Each platform allows a specific number of characters and hashtags allowed in each post. These are the maximum counts to use as a guide, but maximum doesn't mean the best. We also show you, according to platform analytics, how many character counts are the most effective (Table 3-1).

GO TO YOUR AUDIENCE

How do you know where to start or on what platform to focus? Think about your audience from Chapter 2. What is your goal? Whether you are a surgeon, professor, nurse, executive, or resident, thinking about the needs of your audience will help you decide what platforms to use.

DEMOGRAPHICS

New platforms emerge each year and they should always be evaluated for utility to achieving connection with your audience. Knowing the demographics of social media users by platform can be helpful, but don't use it as your only source for determining your primary and secondary audiences. Consider TikTok, for example: If you are a geriatric practitioner and your audience is older adults, you might dismiss TikTok as a relevant platform. However, caregivers of older adults, which could be in any age range over 18 years, may be on TikTok and find your message there because they don't use Facebook. If you were a women's health professional, TikTok might be the most

Table 3-2. Social Media Demographics in the United States

	FACEBOOK	TWITTER	LINKEDIN	INSTAGRAM	YOUTUBE	TIKTOK
U.S. ADULTS	69%	22%	27%	37%	73%	
MEN	63%	24%	29%	31%	78%	40%
WOMEN	75%	21%	24%	43%	68%	60%
WHITE	70%	21%	28%	33%	71%	
BLACK	70%	24%	24%	40%	77%	
HISPANIC	69%	25%	16%	51%	78%	
AGES 18 TO 29 YEARS	79%	38%	28%	67%	91%	62%
30 TO 49 YEARS	79%	26%	37%	47%	87%	30.3%
50 TO 64 YEARS	68%	17%	24%	23%	70%	7.1%
65+ YEARS	46%	7%	11%	8%	38%	

(continued)

useful platform to educate young women about sexual health or answer reproductive questions because 60% of TikTok users are women and 62% are 18 to 29 years old. The primary principle to keep in mind is matching your message to your audience through the platform with the most potential to reach them (Table 3-2).

The Platform Basics

For all platforms, become familiar with the different sections of your account.

Table 3-2. Social Media Demographics in the United States (continued)

	FACEBOOK	TWITTER	LINKEDIN	INSTAGRAM	YOUTUBE	TIKTOK
URBAN	73%	26%	33%	46%	77%	
SUBURBAN	69%	22%	30%	35%	74%	
RURAL	66%	13%	10%	21%	64%	
HIGH SCHOOL OR LESS	61%	13%	9%	33%	64%	
SOME COLLEGE	75%	24%	26%	37%	79%	
COLLEGE+	74%	32%	51%	45%	80%	
<$30,000	69%	20%	10%	35%	68%	
$30,000 TO $74,999	72%	20%	26%	39%	75%	
$75,000	74%	31%	49%	42%	83%	

Adapted from Doyle, B. (2022). TikTok statistics - Updated March 2022. wallaroomedia.com. https://wallaroomedia.com/blog/social-media/tiktok-statistics/; Perrin, A., & Anderson, M. (2019, April 10). Share of US adults using social media, including Facebook, is mostly unchanged since 2018. Pew Research Center. https://pewrsr.ch/2N6Qiht

News Feed

When you sign in to your account, this is the screen that shows up first. It includes all the posts of the people you follow. At first, it might feel frustrating because you can't keep up with and read all the posts. But as you will learn, you're not supposed to. Scan your feed and read, click, like, share, and comment on what you see in that moment. It is almost impossible to read every post from your followers, so just select what is important to you. If you want to see posts from a specific person, you can always go directly to their profile page to see everything you might have missed.

Profile/Timeline

This is your own page—the one that displays your brand. It includes your bio, profile picture, and the posts, shares, tweets, retweets, and likes that you posted directly.

Notifications

This section notifies you if you were tagged, mentioned, or if someone you know liked or commented on a post. Checking your notifications is crucial so you can see who is talking about you and respond appropriately to build your network.

Direct Message

Direct messaging (DM) allows you to send content to individuals privately, much like an email or text. If you are following leaders in your field or journalists, a DM is another way to connect with someone if you don't have their email or phone number. You might also DM with colleagues or friends instead of sending an email. Just remember that although DMs are a way to have a private conversation through your social account, the other person can screenshot your messages and make them public. It is advisable to remember that anything you write online can be discoverable, so don't put anything in writing that you wouldn't want the public, or your supervisor, to see.

What to Do if You Have a Typo

- Facebook lets you edit the post.
- Instagram lets you edit the text but not the photo.
- LinkedIn lets you edit the text but not the photo.
- Twitter does not let you edit tweets, so you have to delete it and repost. However, you may not want to if you already have people engaging with it by posting comments, likes, or retweets. Minor typos are acceptable on Twitter because of this reason so don't worry about being judged by your peers for a spelling error (except in a hashtag) or missing an apostrophe.

WHY TWITTER?

Our rationale for focusing on Twitter is that Twitter has become an influencer marketplace. Almost every industry has a presence on Twitter where professionals are sharing ideas and information. We focus on Twitter for influence because of its design and the millions of active daily users. Many individuals and organizations in the health care industry are already on Twitter having important conversations. The high-speed ability to share and notify others using short form posts and the hashtag (#) function for aggregating topics has emerged as the platform professionals choose to build their networks, amplify their messages, translate health care information for the public, and track the impact of their work.

People are 31% more likely to recall something they see on Twitter compared to general online browsing (Park, 2018). Having a presence on Twitter helps you to articulate the meaning of your work in a digestible manner. Your expertise becomes accessible beyond the walls of the hospital, university, academic journals, and professional organizations. Your practical, real-life knowledge or your research findings or insights on current issues are available for the public and your peers, who are ultimately the people you are trying to reach.

TWITTER BEST PRACTICES

These are the nuts and bolts of Twitter: all the tips, lingo, and tools you need to get started.

Basics of a Tweet

- 280-character limit
- @ are nouns (the account names of people and organizations)
- #hashtags are topics or ideas
- Add a photo or video to your post for more visibility
- Add an article link to your post
- You don't have to be clever, but you should try to be strategic
- Make it easy to scan and read; write your post like you are talking to a non–health care professional
- Make sure to use tags in your post so people can find your topic, but only use one or two hashtags and one or two mentions per post, otherwise your tweet will be hard to read

How to Use Hashtags

Hashtags are the most important concept for Twitter, and all social media channels. Hashtags are the key to connect with people and audiences. To filter through the millions of tweets posted every hour, hashtags help you track conversations about certain topics and ideas. Hashtags are also used to join social movements, relate to cultures and concepts, and express opinions and beliefs.

A hashtag shows up in your post as a different color that is clickable and will take you to a screen with other posts that include the same hashtag. But with only 280 characters available in a tweet, you should not use too many because it makes your post hard to read and ineffective. Strategically choose the best one to two words that contain a popular topic relatable to your post and your audience.

Hashtag Do's and Don'ts

Here are some tips you need to remember when using hashtags in your tweets.

- Do:
  - Keep it short and simple. Only one to two tags per post.
  - Be strategic by using hashtag finder websites. These sites will tell you how many people are using that hashtag, if it is trending, and suggest related hashtags that you might not have considered.
  - Spell check, then check again. You can't edit a post on Twitter, so making sure that your hashtags are spelled correctly is imperative to being effective.
- Don't:
  - Don't make your hashtags more than one to four words. They are hard to read, and you will find most trending hashtags are only one or two words.
  - Don't hashtag every word in your tweet. Not only is this ineffective because not every word in your post deserves a hashtag, but it also makes the post much harder to scan and read.
  - Use a space between hashtags. Make sure there is a space after each word/ phrase that you hashtag. For example, #cardiovascular #hearthealth instead of #cardiovascular#hearthealth.
  - Don't use words that make you unapproachable. Using puffed up words to describe yourself like #guru, #ninja, or #gifted can seem arrogant. Let other people call you these things as a compliment; don't claim them for yourself with a hashtag as this can be harmful to your brand.
  - Don't make typos. The purpose of a hashtag is to connect with others using the same hashtag because in most cases they are interested in the same topics and ideas as you. If you have a typo in your hashtag, it won't be searchable to your prospective community.

80-20 Rule for Content

We recommend adopting an 80-20 rule so that you spend 80% of your time promoting others and 20% of your time on self-promotion. Posting on social media is not your day job, it's a complement to the work you are doing to build your network and reputation. The majority of your posts (80%) should be shares or retweets from other people, your own organization, news sites, and other relevant brands. This type of sharing can be done in a few seconds to a few minutes each day. Once you reach the Create stage, the other 20% of content should be thoughts, ideas, articles, blogs, or other original content created by you. We will share specific ideas about what original content you can post later in the book. This rule not only lessens the amount of time you need to spend on social media, but it also helps build your network. When you share other people's content and tag the post effectively, you are likely to get more followers and engagement. You are creating relationships with people by helping to promote their content. You are also curating the best content for your audience to make things easy to find, which provides value.

Twitter Tools

Lists

Creating lists in Twitter helps you organize the people and organizations that you are following. First, create different categories in your list like "colleagues," "influencers," "news orgs," "journalists," "friends," and "alumni." Then assign the people you follow to one of these categories in the list. Once you start following more than 50 people, your news feed will be filled with their tweets. Creating lists will help you see only the tweets of people in each category. If you want to see what your college alumni connections are talking about, go to the "alumni" list. If you want to see what thought leaders in your industry are talking about, go to the "influencers" list. This filters only the tweets from this list into your news feed. Then switch back and forth as needed.

Mute

When you mute an account, you stay connected to them as a follower, but you won't see their posts in your news feed. This tool is best used when someone's posts are irrelevant, annoying, or clogging up your news feed. You don't want to unfollow them because they are likely to unfollow you back, so muting them is the best option.

Block

If someone is harassing you or there is another reason why you don't want an account to see your public tweets, you can block their account. They will know that you blocked them; if they try to look at your tweets a message will show up saying they were blocked. Block is a feature to use when there is a concern about privacy, safety, or hostility.

Threads

If you have more than 280 characters to share, you can create a Twitter thread. This means you add a label to the end of each tweet such as (1/5), (2/5), etc. Threads should only be used when you 1) have a philosophical argument to make that cannot be explained in one tweet, or 2) want to tell a story that cannot be summed up in one tweet.

HELPFUL HINT: Use a URL Shortener

Since you only have 280 characters on Twitter, it is a waste to use them with long URL article links that you want to share. Shortening the URL will save you characters, and if you sign up for a free bit.ly account, you can even track how many people clicked on your shortened link to read the article or webpage.

HELPFUL HINT: A Word About Emojis

Emojis can be effective on Facebook or Instagram, but we recommend using them sparingly on Twitter and LinkedIn. Your posts will be taken more seriously if you stick to text only in your post, and not follow it up with a smiley face emoji. Also, some emojis are not well known and can be taken in the wrong context. You might occasionally use an emoji in a comment to another person's tweet, especially if it is to congratulate them or if the original post is fun in nature. The full list of emoji names can be found at the Unicode Consortium's website (Unicode Inc, 2020).

FILTER AND FOCUS

Just like an open fire hydrant blasting water onto the street, we are constantly blasted with content from all angles from cell phone alerts and notifications to television programming, billboard ads, and printed mail. But we are especially bombarded from digital channels. Just think about your email inbox—many of us can receive more than 100 messages per day depending on our professional role, and this doesn't include emails from our friends and family.

So much content is available, but you only have a set amount of time to Consume it. People are picky about what they spend their time on, so you need to make your content stand out from the rest.

With so little time and short attention spans, your job is to filter out the most important and interesting content you come across to share with your focused audience.

GETTING STARTED

You know the level at which you are starting on social media. One of the first steps is to create your profile and connect with other people and organizations.

Whether you are new to social media or already have a presence, you can use Table 3-3, and the rest of the book, to determine what you should be doing during each stage of your social media growth.

TABLE 3-3. SOCIAL MEDIA PLATFORMS AND THE 3C's			
	CONSUME	**CONTRIBUTE**	**CREATE**
FACEBOOK	Send friend requests to people you know Read home feed to see what your friends are doing/posting	Like Comment Share Facebook Story Use hashtags in posts	Write posts (use text, photos, graphics, videos) Facebook Live Facebook Events Facebook Page (for business) Facebook Groups Facebook Watch parties
TWITTER	Follow people and organizations that are interesting to you Scan through your news feed to read posts of people you follow Go directly to the accounts of people you follow to keep up with their posts Note the short form style of posts (280 characters or less) What catches your attention?	Like Comment Retweet Retweet with comment DM Use hashtags in posts	Create and follow Twitter Lists Pay attention to your Notifications and to Twitter Analytics
LINKEDIN	Add your education and work history to your profile Connect with people, groups, and organizations that you know Send connection requests to people with shared interests or expertise	Like Comment Share Check your notifications and messages Use hashtags in posts	Write posts Post a video or a document Write a LinkedIn article

(continued)

TABLE 3-3. SOCIAL MEDIA PLATFORMS AND THE 3C'S (CONTINUED)		
	CONSUME	**CONTRIBUTE**	**CREATE**
INSTAGRAM	Follow people Read home feed to see images and videos from the people you are following Watch stories of people you follow	Like Comment Use hashtags in posts	Post images and video to feed and story Use trending hashtags on posts Use stories for more engagement Use IGTV (Instagram TV) for longer videos Add "link in bio" function
YOUTUBE	Search for videos of interest	Subscribe to channels	Create and post videos

REFERENCES

DataReportal. (2022). *Global social media overview*. DataReportal. https://bit.ly/2M4m3ao

Doyle, B. (2022). *TikTok statistics - Updated March 2022*. wallaroomedia.com. https://wallaroomedia.com/blog/social-media/tiktok-statistics/

Gordon, W. (2002, July). *Marshall who? The estate of Corinne & Marshall McLuhan*. https://bit.ly/3nAa7Lp

Jackson, D. (2020, August 3). *Know your limits: The ideal length of every social media post*. Sprout Social. https://bit.ly/2LoPynG

LinkedIn. (2020). *About LinkedIn*. LinkedIn Corporation 2021. https://bit.ly/2KqoiRY

McLuhan, M. (1964). *Understanding media: The extensions of man*. McGraw-Hill.

Osman, M. (2020, December 31). *Mind-blowing LinkedIn statistics and facts (2021)*. Kinsta. https://bit.ly/2XUcIVy

Park, M. (2018, June 12). *Expanding in-stream video ads to more advertisers globally*. Twitter. https://bit.ly/3aBfSEW

Perrin, A., & Anderson, M. (2019, April 10). *Share of US adults using social media, including Facebook, is mostly unchanged since 2018*. Pew Research Center. https://pewrsr.ch/2N6Qiht

Unicode Inc. (2020). *Emoji list, v13.1*. Unicode Emoji Charts. https://bit.ly/3asgCMP

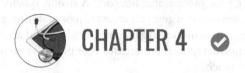

CHAPTER 4 ✅

Using the Fast Lane to Build a Network

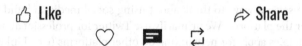

👍 Like   ↪ Share

♡ 💬 ⇄

In the old days, the primary way to meet people was to meet through colleagues or face-to-face at events like conferences. Networking could lead to interesting opportunities—consultations, collaborations, even friendships. This process generally takes years to build a network. But now, with the advent and proliferation of social media, the individuals you would like to know or connect with are only one click away.

Social media is used for building relationships. We've built relationships using social media and you may have too. You know the power of connecting with others who share like interests, from near and far. Connecting with individuals and organizations has never been easier. In the social media world, much like in real life, connecting with people is generally positive. On whatever social media platform(s) you use (e.g., Twitter, LinkedIn), you want to connect to people (and organizations)—you want to follow people and have people follow you (Brooks, 2019). The more followers you have that also follow you the more your chance for influence increases, but it's not just a numbers game.

Shattell, M., Batchelor, M., & Darmoc, R. *Social Media in Health Care: A Guide to Creating Your Professional Digital Presence* (pp. 55-66).
© 2022 Taylor & Francis Group.

Think of it in terms of building your professional network. A strong, quality network is powerful for all kinds of reasons—it can give you access to jobs, publishing and grant opportunities, new colleagues, opportunities to generate new ideas, and access to different information outside your normal sphere. It increases your potential for influence and impact and broadens your reach.

How to Find Organizations and People to Follow

There are several ways to think about using social media to build your network. First, consider the platform. We primarily use Twitter for professional networking, but the same principles apply for networking on other platforms (e.g., LinkedIn).

Organizations

Think about the health care organizations, academic health systems, patient care communities, universities, and community organizations that you admire or whose work somehow intersects with yours. You can go to organizations' websites and search for the social media icons, which are usually at the bottom of the home page. You can easily click on the icons that will take you to the social media accounts and then follow.

Leaders

Look for the leaders and individuals within these organizations and follow them. The main accounts of organizations are often staffed by social media/communications/marketing persons, who are good to connect to, but you also need to find and follow the leaders, editors, and individuals from these organizations. It's through these person-to-person connections, interactions, and engagements that you can find the most opportunities. Look at what the account is retweeting to find people who work at that organization.

Media

Think about journals, magazines, and news sources. Look for these social media accounts the same way, and then follow them. You can also follow the individual accounts of their editors, associate editors, journalists, and writers whom you admire on the organizations' bio pages or directories.

Colleagues and Friends

Search for your coworkers, colleagues, and friends. If you cannot find them, the simplest way is to ask individuals for their social media handles and then follow them. Look for leaders in your own organizations and follow them too. You can use a website such as Followerwonk to search Twitter profiles by topic (Followerwonk, 2020). This is another way to help you find and then follow influencers in your specific field or area of interest.

Friends of Friends

Another way to find and follow people is from the social platform itself. For example, on Twitter, you can go to the account of someone with similar interests, or someone that you know, and then scroll through their list of followers to find individuals and organizations. This strategy can be most effective when you are starting to build your network.

Just Google It

You can use a search engine like Google to find the Twitter handle of someone. Google "What is Mona Shattell's Twitter handle?" to find Mona's Twitter page @MonaShattell in the search results. Click on the link and then follow from the Twitter platform (if you're logged in).

How to Get Others to Follow You

We have several strategies, from simple to more complex. Once you start following people, and others start to follow you, it will be important to engage this new audience. And this goes for all social media platforms.

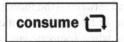

This is the first C—Consume—in our model of social media development. This is the first step in building those whom you follow. For Twitter and other platforms, you start with consuming content—scrolling through your home page and reading what's interesting to you.

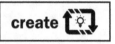

contribute

The second C in our model is Contribute. After you are comfortable consuming, you might start by retweeting the tweets of others. When you retweet with a comment (i.e., quote retweet) and tag others, this allows you to connect with those you follow while building your following.

create

The third C in our model is Create. At this stage you are starting a conversation by creating your own content, sharing your ideas, tagging people and organizations, and using hashtags as a connector to the broader conversation. Consistently producing original content is a quick way to build your following with the public and a global audience.

For building your network, this 3C's Model of Social Media Development offers ways to interest your followers, interact with people and organizations, and influence a conversation by sharing original ideas. Networking allows engagement in the digital social conversations relevant to your expertise.

Twitter Etiquette

Give to Get

The psychology and central theme of expanding your network on Twitter is "give to get." So just like if someone gives you a gift, you feel compelled and sometimes even obligated to give them something back. It's the same theory on Twitter—when someone follows you, follow them back. Most users practice this method, so you will see a return if you do this consistently. This "give to get" approach applies to all your actions on Twitter. The more you give—comments, likes, and retweets—the more you will get back in return, and the more it will keep you engaged and wanting to do more. Checking your notifications on Twitter will help you know when someone engaged with your content or followed you, so that you can engage back.

TIPS TO BUILD YOUR FOLLOWING

Public Profiles

We suggest that you do all that you can to make your social media profiles more visible. This means making your Twitter profile "public" rather than "private" in your settings. The goal is to limit any barriers to connecting with other professionals. Only keep the privacy settings to private for your personal social media accounts.

Integrate Social

We recommend that you add your Twitter (and other platform) handles on your business cards, in your email signature lines, university/agency websites, on PowerPoint presentations—and for those in higher education, include social in your course syllabi.

What's Your Handle?

When you meet people face-to-face, ask to connect via social media. This is the new way to make lasting connections and may eventually replace asking for business cards that then get lost or simply pile up in desk drawers, and therefore never result in further communication. Once you are connected via social, it's a much easier and more sustainable relationship.

CONFERENCE CONNECTIONS

You can use social media before, during, and after scholarly, academic, or clinical conferences to connect with others in your field.

Before You Go

The most important networking and visibility tool is the conference hashtag. Many times the conference hashtag is listed on conference websites and brochures, but if it is not, you may need to email or tweet to the organization or ask a friend. Conference hashtags are important because they bring people together so others can follow what's happening at the conference. For example, whether one is a conference goer or not, anyone can follow the social media posts of a conference if they have the hashtag, and if people who tweet from the conference use it.

If you are presenting at a conference, as you prepare your presentation, consider including your Twitter handle and conference hashtag on each slide. You might also add suggested hashtags to each slide, or sample tweets.

Use the conference hashtag in a pre-conference tweet (e.g., "Looking forward to #Academy2020 when 5 of my @hopkinsnursing colleagues will be inducted into the @AAN_Nursing tomorrow!"). Before you go, or when you are on the way, or when you arrive, you could tweet "Excited to attend #Academy2020 to see @nursingdean." This is a good opportunity to use images (e.g., at the airport).

You have created your presentation and included your twitter handle and conference hashtag on your poster or slides, sent one or two pre-conference tweets, and are now ready when you arrive, or when the conference starts.

During the Conference

This is when most of the social media engagement will happen—it's prime time for networking. But you will have prepared for it beforehand. You are connecting with others. Some of you might remember the old days when on-site conferences would have a "message board." Attendees could post little pieces of paper on the board for individual attendees to make connections and meet. Now, you can use social media and Twitter to do the same thing, and it's more efficient. When you tag/mention someone in a tweet or send them a direct message (DM), you can be almost sure they will see it; unlike wondering if they happened to walk by the message board and see your note.

The notes on the message board, or the tweets and DMs, are usually to people whom you already know; however, Twitter and DMs can also be used during conferences to get to know new people. These are people whom we might not have known before but we will now follow. We like, retweet, and sometimes tag them in tweets. We "get to know them" through their tweets and may ask to meet them #IRL (in real life) during the conference to follow up on shared interests. When we attend conferences, or even if we are not at the conference but are following along on Twitter, we look for who is tweeting. These "chance" meetings through your use of the conference hashtag can result in opportunities down the road.

Live Tweeting

Write tweets of pithy content heard in presentations, and tag presenters in your tweets (and add the conference hashtag, of course), and other relevant hashtags. If the presenter talks about something that is similar or somehow relates to your own work, say so in a tweet, and add a link or an image to your work. Again, you are using social media to build connections.

Pictures and Videos

Take pictures and short videos at the conference and tag those who are in them. Search for Twitter handles of keynotes and other presenters (which, of course, should be on their slides but often is not), and follow them. Comment on the presentations and content.

Chatbox

For virtual conferences, you might also connect with others by using the video conferencing chatbox, and ask others to share their Twitter handle, or you can even rename yourself/profile name to your Twitter handle.

Presenting

If you are a presenter at an in-person conference, you might want to pass around an old-fashioned sign-in sheet to gather Twitter handles of all your session participants, which you can then follow later, or create a list in Twitter. This allows you to create continued connections by following audience members and encouraging them to follow each other. You can also pre-schedule your own tweets (e.g., use Hootsuite) to go out during your presentation, and then your colleagues can live tweet during your session.

Conference Apps

Many conferences these days use conference apps, which you can and should use to create a profile and include your Twitter handle. Conference-goers can then have another way to access you and your social media accounts. Think about your professional brand and be sure that your profile in the conference app is consistent with this brand.

After the Conference

Although most of the tweeting will stop, it's good to now take a few minutes to review your social media presence. Check out your Twitter analytics to see how much engagement you had and how many new followers you've gained. See what content generated the most interest and send follow-up tweets and DMs to your new connections.

KEEP YOUR SOCIAL MEDIA PROFILES UP TO DATE

Profiles Matter

Your Twitter profile (and your profiles on all social media platforms) is important, and can always be improved. A better profile can lead to more and better connections, and greater amplification. You want your profile to represent your professional brand.

We suggest that you review your social media profiles across platforms every few months, or more frequently, and update information and images as appropriate. Think of your profile like you would your curriculum vitae or résumé. It should be updated and truly reflect who you are today. Also, we have found that a little tweak in your profile could have dramatically positive results (more engagement from others). Thus, don't be afraid to try out different phrases, handles, hashtags, and tones in your bio. It's easy to change back again if you find that a newly revised profile isn't working as well as you had hoped.

ON BEING TWITTER-VERIFIED

The Blue Checkmark

"Twitter-Verified" is the blue checkmark that you see next to an individual or organization's Twitter handle. Being verified on Twitter means that Twitter has checked to see that you are who you say you are and given you the blue checkmark. Most often, Twitter verification is reserved for those who are celebrities, politicians, athletes, activists, or those considered "influential." This is because fake accounts are created for celebrities that make it difficult to know which account belongs to the actual celebrity. In the past, Twitter had a process that allowed individuals and businesses to apply to be Twitter-Verified, but they discontinued this process a few years ago. As of 2022, Twitter implemented a new verification process. We suggest that you follow @verified to stay up to date with the current verification process. You might ask, how many followers does it take to get verified? This does not seem to be the key factor—some people have gotten verified with relatively few followers, others with many more, but again, follow @verified on Twitter for current information.

How to Use Hashtags and Handles to Engage Others

Using hashtags and handles is how amplification and connection works; they leverage the power of social media and accelerate building your professional network.

Hashtags

Hashtags started with Twitter but are now being used across platforms. When composing a tweet, a good rule of thumb is to include at least one handle (person or organization) and one hashtag (an idea). As you may recall, a hashtag is the number sign (#) and it brings together ideas or concepts. This is how communities build, form relationships, and connect with each other (e.g., #MentalHealth, #Aging, #SocialMedia, #Marketing). If you are interested in any of these topics, you can type it in the search bar in Twitter and see who is tweeting or writing about that specific topic. This is important because it can help you stay up to the minute with conversations and happenings related to your topics of interest, and it can help you to identify new followers. To engage others, it helps by connecting your tweet to a larger audience.

Tagging With Hashtags

Do you create your own or use hashtags that others create? Hashtags are only useful if they are intuitive to others or if others are already using them. So, this is a time when you don't want to be too creative, because if you are, others may not find you or the topic. For example, a not-so-good hashtag could be "#ImGoingToItaly" but a good one could be "#ItalyTravel." In our field of health care, you can use a website such as the Symplur Healthcare Hashtag Project, a live repository of current health care–related hashtags that is available without cost (Symplur, 2020). It is crowdsourced as well, so if you want to add a hashtag (e.g., a conference hashtag or other) to their list, you can submit a request. Another website and free service is RiteTag, which suggests hashtags with statistics on their usage, and populates related hashtags to help you decide the best ones to use (RiteTag, 2020). For hashtags in general, to be clear, you can use hashtags that are not listed on Symplur or suggested by RiteTag or any other website or social media platform, but you should use hashtags that others are using as well.

Finding Conference Hashtags

You can also use Symplur to find and follow conferences that are trending, so that you can follow along and engage with conference-goers in the moment (Symplur, 2020). You don't have to attend the conference to be able to participate and create high engagement with the conference hashtag, tweets, and the individuals tweeting from the conference. Conference hashtags must be used in your posts when tweeting about the conferences because the hashtag galvanizes people around the event.

Handles

It's important to use handles, which "tag" a person or an organization because they are somehow related to what you are tweeting. Tagging a person using their handle triggers a notification to them. It lets the person or organization know that someone has mentioned them. It brings your tweet to their direct attention—to their "inbox" so to speak.

Tagging With Handles

Think of tagging someone with their handle as cc'ing them. And this can be used to increase your reach and connect others to your tweets.

Twitter Tips to Increase Engagement

Initial Post

You build engagement by incorporating #hashtags and @handles in your tweets. If you know of a colleague who published a recent paper, you can tweet about the paper being published in a journal such as the *Journal of Psychosocial Nursing and Mental Health Services* (@JPNJournal). Include the @handle of the author and their organization (Dr. Catherine Ling [@CGLingPhDFNP], Johns Hopkins School of Nursing [@HopkinsNursing]) with an image/graphic. Include other key #hashtags to alert readers to the focus of the paper. In this instance, the paper was about suicide, so #suicide was added to the tweet. The #hashtag allows connection with others who are interested in the topic of suicide and the @handles alert the author and the organization of the post.

Response

After Dr. Ling saw the tweet (because she was tagged), she retweeted it and added a tag of someone who was instrumental in the piece.

How Engaging With Others on Twitter Increases Your Network

Twitter Engagement

You can and should tag others and use hashtags in your tweets, but also, think about how else you can further your engagement. You can participate and organize Twitter chats and Twitter conferences such as Nursing Mutual Aid 2020 (2020) #NMA2020, which are chats and conferences held exclusively on Twitter—free and open to the public.

Twitter Chats

Twitter chats are planned before a main event and typically occur the hour before the main event online. Twitter chats are essentially focused, digital conversations on a certain topic; using a particular hashtag so others can follow along; allow for a prepared and timed discussion/engagement questions; and a subsequent discussion. Twitter chats are a good way to connect with more people with similar interests. Think of it as an online meet-up to discuss a topic of mutual interest, with persons from all across the globe.

Are Twitter Notifications and Analytics Important?

Short answer—YES. The easiest way to increase your engagement on Twitter is to routinely check your notifications. Twitter has several built-in notifications and analytics systems, and we recommend using them. They help you pay attention to your followers and engagement levels. Which posts do your followers retweet and comment on? This tells you what content is most interesting to your followers.

Notifications

Twitter notifies you (in the app) when someone mentions you, comments, or likes your content. It's important for you to keep up with this so that you can respond. Your new followers will be listed here, as well as any comments, and all the people who liked your posts. When you review your notifications, you can also get a sense of which content is most engaging to your followers. Remember: "Give to Get."

Analytics

Analytics for Twitter are available in the app and gives you a snapshot of your activity and engagement (from your home screen, click on "More" and then "Analytics"). You get a past 28-day summary with a percent change from the previous month: 1) the total number of tweets that you posted, 2) the total number of tweet impressions (total number of times a tweet was seen), 3) the total number of times someone visited your profile, 4) the total number of times someone mentions you on Twitter, and 5) the total number of followers with a number of increase (or decrease) from the following month. You also will see your top tweet, top follower (with the most followers), and top mention.

Analytics Rule of Thumb

We think it's important to at least view your Twitter analytics once per month, or more frequently, to help you know what your audience is responding to and help you tailor your media presence to build your network.

REFERENCES

Brooks, B. A. (2019). LinkedIn and your professional identity. *Nurse Leader, 17*(3), 173-175. https://doi.org/10.1016/j.mnl.2019.03.001

Followerwonk. (2020). *Search bios.* https://followerwonk.com/bio/

Nursing Mutual Aid. (2020). *#NMA2020 conference archive.* NursingMutualAid.SquareSpace.com. https://bit.ly/3pR3zZT

Ritetag. (2020). *No idea what hashtags to use?* https://ritetag.com

Symplur. (2020). *Healthcare hashtag project.* https://bit.ly/2LLEhNP

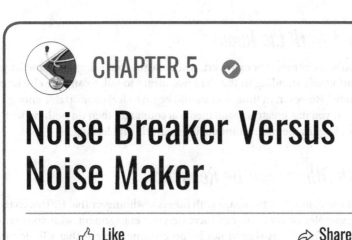

CHAPTER 5 ✅

Noise Breaker Versus Noise Maker

👍 Like   ➥ Share

♡ 💬 ⇄

> "Social media is the ultimate equalizer.
> It gives a voice and a platform to anyone willing to engage."
>
> *Amy Jo Martin*
> *@AmyJoMartin*

SETTING EXPECTATIONS

Would you just walk into a cocktail party, loudly announce that you have arrived, and then leave the room? Probably not. Particularly since the point of attending the cocktail party is more than just making an entrance—the main point is to engage with other people. For the extroverts in the world, these types of interactions may come naturally.

What About Introverts?

Many introverts would avoid social events like a cocktail party, but would have more confidence to interact in a controlled environment. Interacting via social media gives a person more time to think about the level and type of engagement they wish to have and think through what they want to say ahead of time. This takes the pressure off introverts and has the potential to level the playing field for networking and building your professional presence.

Shattell, M., Batchelor, M., & Darmoc, R. *Social Media in Health Care:*
A Guide to Creating Your Professional Digital Presence (pp. 67-90).
© 2022 Taylor & Francis Group.

Show Up and Work the Room

Whether you're an introvert or extrovert, when starting out using social media you may only be comfortable standing in the shadows, afraid to talk to anyone else or put anything "out there." However, in time, you should begin to feel comfortable enough to "work the room." If you just create a social media account and then do nothing with it, that's a lot like walking in the room, announcing yourself, and leaving.

Engage With Others, But Be Realistic

The point of social media is to engage with others—whomever that is. This chapter contains many examples of how you can increase your engagement with your target audience over time. Your focus should not be on creating content that will go viral; instead, your focus should be on serving a core group of 1000 followers. When your goal is building up to 1000 people who are interested in the health information (and/ or other content) that you are sharing, it mentally takes a lot of pressure off you. It's unrealistic to think that any (or all) of your posts will go viral.

NOISE MAKERS AND NOISE BREAKERS

Making noise is critical because remaining silent doesn't change anything. If you only Consume social media, you are silent and invisible—and maybe that's your comfort level or it's appropriate for the time, energy, and context of what you are consuming. You can make occasional Contributions, but you don't have to comment on everything. Only being a Noise Maker isn't a good or bad thing; in fact, sometimes making a lot of noise is an excellent strategy for moving an agenda or social movement forward.

What's the Difference?

The Noise Makers of the world will get attention, but evolving to a Noise Breaker is a subtle shift that puts you in a leadership role whatever the conversation. You begin providing your unique perspective/thought leadership capacity. You Create the conversation and engage with others to amplify your message. There are likely certain times and places where you need to be one or the other, or both. It's up to you to know and understand how to use the power of both to get your message out there and amplify it with your target audience.

The Art of the Zigzag

It is most likely that you will move back and forth between being a Noise Maker and a Noise Breaker as you zigzag your way to making an impact through social media.

At the Contribute level, you can add to the noise by retweeting and sharing to amplify the messages of others. This is also fine, but if you don't add a comment, your voice won't be heard. Only sharing what everyone else is posting without adding your voice and unique perspective limits the conversation.

Upping Your Game

Our goal is to help you to be strategic with upping your game to the level of being a more consistent Noise Breaker. By actively engaging with your followers (audience), you build relationships over time and establish your thought leadership in your area of expertise. What follows are strategies to keep in mind as you embark on your social media journey.

PERSUASIVE MESSAGING

With content bombarding us from all angles, it's no wonder some people feel overwhelmed when thinking about adopting social media. But those who use it effectively and have the most impact know a secret. It's something strategic communicators and journalists use in almost all communication decisions: how to persuade someone with the fewest number of words in the shortest amount of time.

Our attention spans have changed since our world became digital. We scan instead of read from beginning to end (Carr, 2020). As social media users scan through news feeds, what will make your message stand out from the rest? Later on, we discuss different ways to hone your core message. Once you have identified your core message, you then need to think about how to best frame it.

IDENTIFYING YOUR CORE MESSAGE

Half-Life Your Message

We all have multiple things competing for our attention. The fastest way to lose your audience is to take too long to get to your point. One tool to get to your core message with any communication is to "Half-Life Your Message." Originally used in improvisational theater, this tool has been adapted to help academic writers and presenters learn how to communicate more effectively (Aurbach et al., 2018). In 3 minutes, you repeatedly shorten the same message in order to practice idea prioritization. Using a timer that you can see, start talking out loud about your topic of interest for 60 seconds, then repeat the process with only 30 seconds to convey your message, then in 15 seconds, and a final round with only 8 seconds to convey your core message. While this exercise is intended to be completed with a partner, you can also try this by yourself by recording your answers using the Memo app on your iPhone or recording a video.

Use a Message Box

Once you have identified your core message, you can use the Message Box tool to identify supporting themes and related talking points that may have been eliminated in the "Half-Life Your Message" exercise (Aurbach et al., 2018). Developed by COMPASS, the Message Box helps communicators define the problem, solution, benefits, and significance of their topic of interest in a written format (COMPASS Science Communications Inc., 2017).

FRAMING YOUR CORE MESSAGE

Maslow Needs + Twitter

Maslow's Hierarchy of Needs is more than just a psychological model for meeting human needs. It can also help you theoretically think through how to best deliver your message. This model is often used throughout the marketing cycle to develop a brand strategy and frame communications, based on consumer behavior research (Figure 5-1). Most corporate brands focus their messaging on the top three tiers to create loyalty with their customers. But for article headlines or Twitter posts, any of the top four work well.

Framing the Message

Crafting communications with underlying needs and values connects a person emotionally to your message and makes them want to know more. Think of your posts as teasers that hit on one of these needs. Using Maslow's Hierarchy of Needs is a key component of catching the attention and increasing the engagement of your audience with your original content model.

Effective Framing

You're at the grocery checkout line where you only have time to scan the magazine titles, and there is a limited amount of time for you to decide whether you want to pick one up and make a purchase. The best examples to learn from are newsstand magazines because this experience mirrors people's online behavior and attention spans. The messages on the cover are essential and you'll notice that they hit on deeper psychological needs that we all have: being in the know, being prepared, feeling safe, feeling loved, or having a sense of belonging and purpose.

It's the same with articles shared on social—is your post easy and interesting enough for someone scanning through it to click on the article and read it? And more importantly, will they react to your post with a like, comment, or retweet? First, take notice of what article links you personally click on to get information. Is it because the headline or tweet appeals to one of your higher-level needs? Craft your messages to align with an audience need, but make sure it is based on the content of the article.

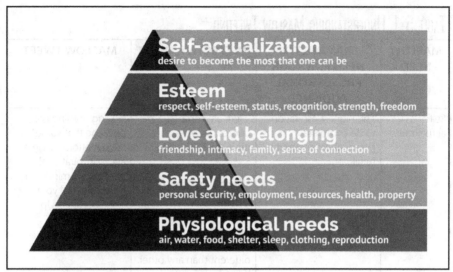

Figure 5-1. Maslow's Hierarchy of Needs. (Plateresca/shutterstock.com)

Application

Whether you are promoting your own article with a tweet or retweeting someone else's content with a comment of your own, understanding the difference between in-effective messages and Maslow messages is essential for success in our 3C's Model of Social Media Development (Table 5-1).

Adjusting Tone and Style

Social media requires you to be open minded in adopting a new tone and writing style in order to make your knowledge accessible and interesting to a non-academic audience. Tone usually refers to how a writer uses certain words in a specific way to convey non-verbal observations about specific subjects. Not only does tone help to deliver facts, but it delivers them with an attitude and emotion. Social media posts are informal writing—don't use scientific abbreviations or jargon; contractions are okay. References are not needed.

Persuasive Video

Core Message First

Most people also stop watching videos after a few seconds—in fact, it's been re-ported that 47% of a video's value is delivered in the first 3 seconds (O'Neill, 2020). Clearly stating your primary message up front will determine whether or not viewers will continue to listen/watch. Keep in mind that you will lose 33% of viewers after 30 seconds, 45% by 1 minute, and 60% by 2 minutes (Bitable, 2020).

TABLE 5-1. UNDERSTANDING MASLOW TWEETING

MASLOW NEED	FRAMING THE NEED FOR YOUR PROFESSIONAL AUDIENCE	INEFFECTIVE TWEET	MASLOW TWEET
Self-actualization	The highest aspiration to be complete, personal growth and fulfillment.	"Here are some good quotes on White privilege." **Why this isn't best:** It doesn't break through all the other posts on privilege; it doesn't say why this article is different than any other. What makes them "good" quotes?	"Saying nothing is a privilege that some are not afforded. Here are 10 inspirational quotes to remind you how powerful your voice is. #SpeakUp #BeTheChange"
Esteem	Lead the pack, be in the know and ahead of the game. Be respected. These are also things you can talk about at a dinner party to start an interesting conversation.	"Read my latest article on naloxone." **Why this isn't best:** How does this relate to me? It doesn't tell me why I should care or pay attention.	"Carrying #naloxone can be the difference between life & death. Read my article @huffpost and learn how you can make a difference."
Love and belonging	Being part of the group, joining others—fellow educators, professionals, clinicians in your industry. Or connecting with friends by congratulating them on an important achievement.	"Interesting article..." **Why this isn't best:** This tells me nothing about the article and I don't have time to figure out if what you find interesting is also interesting to me.	"Nurse Practitioners: here are the top three things you need to know about #automation and the future of #healthcare. Via @healthtechnews"

(continued)

Optimize for Sound Off

The majority of videos are watched without sound—up to 85% of the time (O'Neill, 2020). You need to include text with your audiovisual product, otherwise, the message will be lost.

TABLE 5-1. UNDERSTANDING MASLOW TWEETING (CONTINUED)			
MASLOW NEED	**FRAMING THE NEED FOR YOUR PROFESSIONAL AUDIENCE**	**INEFFECTIVE TWEET**	**MASLOW TWEET**
Safety needs	Think in terms of the body, health, and not putting yourself in physical harm or risk. From a professional view: don't put your career at risk by missing something that's trending or on the horizon for your area of practice.	"Read this new article about food." **Why this isn't best:** It doesn't peak my interest about how this affects my safety, should be concerning to my health, or how to avoid associated danger.	"Possible carcinogen found in a common #heartburn medication is present in some foods. Find out which ones to avoid in my @sciam article."
Physiological needs	This level is based on basic human needs and messaging wouldn't have an emotional component; it is about basic survival. Therefore, this level is not typically included in persuasive messaging—as if you needed connection to a food pantry or homeless shelter, those types of messages fall under Safety Needs (resources).		

Closed Captioning

Be sure to include closed captioning and words that show up within the video. This is also best practice for accessibility.

Within Facebook

You can also add captions to your videos on Facebook by uploading your video as a draft and editing the video to include captions (Salshutz, 2017).

Use iMovie

You can also add titles or insert images with text (e.g., save a PowerPoint slide as a .jpeg and insert as a photo within your video) using iMovie from your phone or desktop.

Optimize for Mobile

Most people access social media from a mobile device (O'Neill, 2020). Preview your content on a mobile device to make sure the images work and text is legible.

Optimal Video Length

Keep your video as short as possible. Your goal for social media videos is to capture attention through a "teaser" video that leads followers to your long-form content on your website, YouTube Channel, Facebook, or LinkedIn. Long-form videos posted to YouTube are ideally 6 to 8 minutes (O'Neill, 2020). Short-form, teaser videos shared on social media can be framed as content teasers for your blog, video, or course; offer a sneak peek to build anticipation for new content or a new product; or be framed as a service teaser by posing a question to those who may be interested in your product or service (Animoto, 2020).

Twitter

Videos on Twitter can be 20 seconds to 2 minutes (to match its character limit), but ideally you will want to keep these videos to 30 seconds or shorter (O'Neill, 2020).

Instagram

Videos on the Instagram feed can be up to 1 minute in length, but videos that are an average of 26 seconds receive the most comments (O'Neill, 2020). Instagram Stories can be up to 15 seconds or you can post multiple 15-second videos to convey your message.

How to Develop Technical Skills

If you are already an educator, Apple Teacher is a program we highly recommend (Apple Inc., 2020). Through this free, online program, you complete six badges for Mac or iPad to learn how to use applications such as iMovie, Keynote, GarageBand, and more. If you are not an educator, you can also attend free, in-person sessions at your nearest Apple Store through the Apple Store app. And if that's not convenient, search YouTube to find tutorials on how to do pretty much anything else.

Flip Your Traditional Work

Think about ways to translate traditional publications and/or presentation content into different formats to expand your reach. For example, record a traditional lecture with PowerPoint using audio or video, and post it. This will move your work from only reaching the audience in the room on that particular day to making it available online for others to benefit.

Flip

For a traditional lecture on "How a Bill Becomes a Law," you can turn it into a short 2-minute video for students taking a health policy course and post it to YouTube (Batchelor, 2019b). You can flip any traditional lecture in PowerPoint or Keynote (allows you to create movement within a presentation) by adding an audio recording (narrated presentation). The presentation can then be imported into iMovie to add music if you would like. By posting it to YouTube, the resource is now publicly available to other faculty to use who are teaching the same content.

Chunk Content

Be sure to think through how much content to include in any new format. If you used 34 slides for a traditional 1-hour presentation, you need to break the content down into smaller "chunks." Rather than cramming all of the content into one long podcast, create a series and break the content down into digestible segments for viewers/listeners.

Flip + Chunk

For a traditional 1-hour presentation on Alzheimer's disease, it would not be difficult to cover three topics such as the warning signs, the diagnostic process, and communication tips. To communicate most effectively using social media, focus on one core message per video. Create three shorter, 15-minute presentations such as the 10 Warning Signs of a Memory Problem, Six Tips for Talking to Someone You Think May Have a Memory Problem, and How Alzheimer's Is Diagnosed will be more effective (Batchelor, 2020c, 2020e, 2020f).

Develop Multiple Assets

Think through how to create multiple assets for your content. In the previous example, the podcast was also developed into a blog and posted on a website. The audio and audiovisual version of the podcast was also posted to the same page and on YouTube. The audiovisual podcast was even broken down into three short, 30- to 60-second clips called microcontent.

Flip + Chunk + Microcontent

If your original content is long-form (over 3 minutes), you can create shorter clips (30 to 60 seconds) known as microcontent to capture attention (Sellas, 2020). You can also create a graphic with a quote or meme that highlights some aspect of your original content. Microcontent posted on social media is a good way to attract your audience's attention and direct those who are interested in learning more by linking the social media posts to the original long-form content. Creating multiple types of assets that can be posted to social media outlets gives you more variety in the ways in which you engage with your audience.

Then What?

Share it with a broader audience. Develop a media and social media implementation plan around the audiovisual microcontent to post across multiple platforms (Twitter, Instagram, LinkedIn, and Facebook). The audio versions can be posted on your website, but also posted to multiple podcast platforms (e.g., iTunes, Stitcher, Amazon Music, Spotify). This allows you to grow a diverse group of followers based on the platforms they already use, even if you don't use the platforms personally.

SKILLS FOR ADDING VALUE
TO THE CONVERSATION

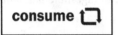

Monitoring the Conversations on Social Media

This the perfect way to get started using social media. When you see posts by others, you can like/share/retweet content that you support (or oppose) to help amplify the noise around an issue. This can be important in getting the attention of the media or policymakers when a lot of noise is being made about an issue and can result in change.

Social Media Influencing Policy

An example of how a social media campaign may have influenced health policy is the BOLD Alzheimer's Act ("BOLD Infrastructure for Alzheimer's Act," 2018; Figure 5-2). When this legislation was introduced in 2017 to the 115th Congress, the Alzheimer's Association and Alzheimer's Impact Movement gave the legislation a hashtag on social media: #BOLDAlzheimersAct. These organizations continue to use the hashtag to keep the public up to date on its progress through the appropriations process (Alzheimer's Impact Movement, 2020). It's also highly likely that the hashtag will be used throughout the implementation process as well.

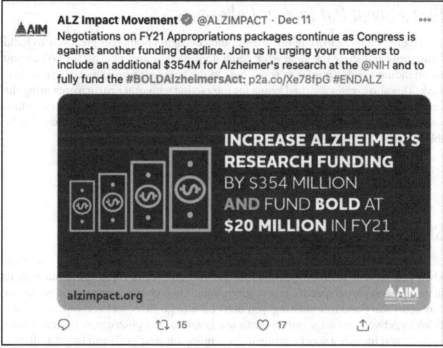

Figure 5-2. Social media raising awareness of legislation. (Reproduced with permission from Alzheimer's Impact Movement, 2020.)

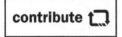

Share Industry and/or Company News

Many people are getting news and announcements through their social media channels these days. Being "in the know" and being willing to share what comes across your desk each day is another great way to engage with your audience. Passing along a newly published journal article, textbook, or research finding is another way to establish your expertise. In addition to sharing news to keep others up to date, consider adding a question (or a poll) about the shared news that followers can chime in and engage with as well as your content.

Highlight Your Organization

Has your organization done something amazing that they have posted on social media or in a newsletter? Passing along information in your world to consumers and/or stakeholders in your area is another great way to highlight the work of your organization. If your organization is embedded in another social media entity, talk with leadership to create an identifiable social media presence specifically for you.

Give a Shout Out to Your Colleagues

Highlighting the work of our friends and colleagues is another great way to build community and share the great work being done in your area of expertise. When you are attending a webinar, give a "shout out" to the speaker to bring awareness to their work. This also creates a virtual venue for interacting with other participants using the same hashtags/handles. Also, when you find a "life hack" that works for you within your brand, you can share those suggestions, tips, and tricks that others may also be able to use.

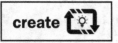

Share Your Unique Perspective

We get to the level of Create by upping our game by at least making a comment when you retweet or share information from others. Think creatively about how to share your unique perspective on any given topic. Own your expertise—and while this may seem scary and intimidating, you don't have to go "live" on Facebook or create a video to get your message out, you can use graphics or a photograph to depict your message and include a short comment. Depending on your goals and target audience, create short- and/or long-form content in a format that works best for you and your message.

Engage With Thought Leaders

If you know an expert who has a unique insight into the field or current event, engage that person by asking them to answer a question on Twitter, write a guest blog, or agree to be interviewed. You can also create a social media post highlighting the work and voice of the expert if you don't have time to arrange anything more complicated.

GETTING AND KEEPING YOUR AUDIENCE'S ATTENTION

People remember visual information six times longer than anything they read or hear. Our brains need an average of 60 seconds to understand 200 to 250 words; understanding an image takes one-tenth of a second. You can increase your views up to 94% by adding a relevant image (Tamble, 2019). Creating videos is the future—social video generates 12 times the shares than text and images combined (Mansfield, 2020; Templeman, 2017).

Therefore, as you develop more advanced social media skills, you will need to think about developing a content strategy that includes video, images, and graphics.

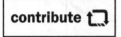

Getting Attention

There are a few different ways to think about content:

- Responding to current events with your unique perspective
- Reposting prior content linked to a current event or conference topic
- Generating content ahead of time for both the traditional and non-traditional/ seasonal calendars (Holidays Calendars, n.d.)

Graphics + Graphic Apps

The use of an image, either a picture or graphic, will help increase engagement with your content and social media posts. They are no longer optional; they are an essential part of a successful social media strategy. Tweets with images average a 150% increase in retweets (Tamble, 2019). Another unique way to Contribute to the conversation is to create a graphic or infographic. You can use free apps on your phone or iPad such as WordSwag, Canva, or Unsplash.

Wordswag

With WordSwag (free or can upgrade to a Pro Package), you can use a photo from your camera, your photo library, or use free stock photos from the app. You can add text for your messaging (Oringe, 2020). Even something as simple as turning a quote into a graphic can see an average of a 19% boost in retweets (@smfrogers, 2014).

Canva

With Canva (also free or you can upgrade to Canva Pro), you can design a visual for your Instagram or Facebook Post or an Instagram Story; or you can create logos, posters, invitations, photo collages, blog graphics, or infographics (Canva Pty Ltd, 2020). With the infographic feature, you can choose from several templates and visually communicate your message in a unique way. You can turn a presentation into an infographic easily using this app (Figure 5-3).

Unsplash

Unsplash is an app that allows you access to free stock photos that can be used to add a photo to your social media posts and/or presentations (Unsplash Inc, 2020). For example, when covering a hearing by the United States Senate Special Committee on Aging, the expert testifying was sharing tips for aging well. Tweeting the tips with a stock photo made the post more interesting than a photo of the back of the expert's head from a seat in the audience (Figure 5-4).

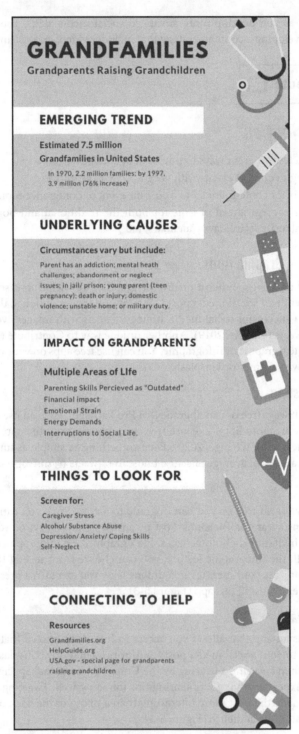

Figure 5-3. Flipping a presentation into an Infographic.

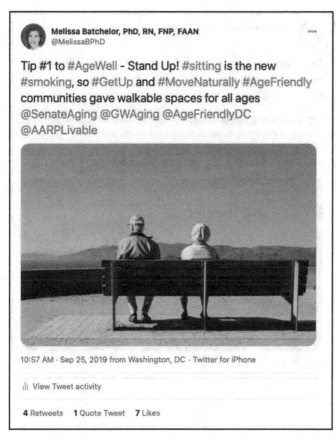

Figure 5-4. Tweet using image from Unsplash (Batchelor, 2019c).

Post Images

Prior to or during a presentation, you can take a photo and tag co-authors. This also allows them to retweet your content (Figure 5-5).

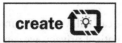

Answer Common Questions

Depending on your area of expertise, record a short video to answer a common question. Search engine optimization allows searchers to search in the form of questions. You can search YouTube to see what the most common questions are in your field and record a short video to answer them.

Figure 5-5. Retweeting a slide presentation (Batchelor, 2019a).

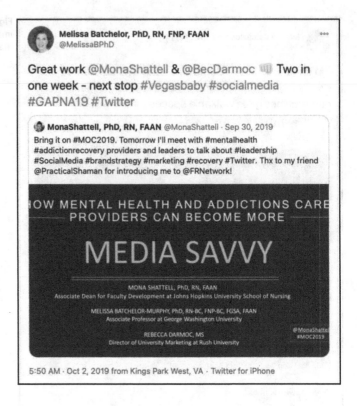

Storytelling

Using a story or case study is one strategy for pulling emotion into your content to make it more memorable. You can also combine this strategy with giving your audience "three things to know." Weaving in a story/case study is a great way to engage your audience in a way that's teachable, memorable, and "sticky."

Sharing Your Stories

As health care professionals, we have stories that only we can tell. We have a unique perspective. While observing all of the rules of HIPAA and patient privacy, we can still create stories or a case study to highlight a current event in a unique way that most often will illuminate the human side of whatever the discussion is about (e.g., children being separated from parents at the border, nurses' experiences during COVID-19). The public and journalists are hungry for these types of stories.

Self-Publish or Mainstream Media

For this longer form of original content, you can write a blog or op-ed, and either self-publish or submit to a news outlet. If self-publishing, the best choices in platform would be on your own professional website, Facebook, or LinkedIn. For any of these long-form posts, be sure to create a short-form post that fits Twitter and Instagram requirements and provide the link to your content to reach your audiences on those platforms.

"Behind the Scenes" Content

If you are hosting an event or a conference, take photos of those helping to set up and send these out via social media as "behind the scenes" content to get your audience excited about attending or intrigued enough to want to join you.

RipL

To make this more visually interesting, you can use the RipL app (free version) to turn photos into a short 10-second video clip (Ripl Inc., 2020). Created on your iPhone, choose a Ripl template, upload photos, and create your captions. Then post to Facebook, Instagram, LinkedIn, Twitter, or YouTube to share your message (Batchelor, 2017).

Show People How It's Done

Based on your area of expertise, rather than writing out how to do something, think about the value of a tutorial, a video that shows people how to do something.

Video Demonstration

YouTube is a powerful search engine for finding exactly that. Given that most people are visual learners, a demonstration video is always a winner if done well. If an activity is complex and difficult to articulate in writing, create a demonstration video (Batchelor-Murphy, 2019). AARP has an entire Family Caregiver How-To Video series born out of the Home Alone Alliance report. These videos demonstrate basic caregiving and nursing skills and medical tasks for family caregivers; it can be simple things that you think everyone should know. For example, Melissa used this strategy in a podcast about "Taking Care of Yourself if You Are Sick" to demonstrate how to fold your bedding in such a way that the least amount of effort is needed to pull your covers up if you have a fever with chills. Rather than just telling people how to do this, seeing it done really brings the point home.

Record Your Screen

You can record your screen to demonstrate the steps in a process. This is particularly helpful when you have provided written instructions for the steps but continue to get questions from others. For example, if you have written out instructions for students to navigate an online course, you will save everyone time by just recording your screen and visually walking the person through the process rather than replying in a written format (that they didn't understand in the first place!). On a laptop, you can use Zoom, Jing, or other programs to record your screen and share the .mp4 file.

How to Screen Record on an iPhone or iPad

If you are using your iPhone or an iPad, you can record your screen by adding the Screen Recording function to your Control Center. Go to Settings > Control Center > and add Screen Recording. This will allow you to quickly access Screen Recording from your Home Screen by swiping down, and selecting Screen Recording. Be sure you turn on your microphone and record. The Screen Recording is saved as a video in your Photos. Share as you normally would share a video (now wouldn't this process make for a great tutorial video?!;Tech Insider, 2018).

Be Inspirational

If part of your brand is to be inspirational, you can use WordSwag or Canva to take an inspirational quote and turn it into an image that can be posted on your social media platform.

Top 3, 5, or 10 Lists

People love lists and checklists! When creating content, think about how to develop a list of helpful hints, strategies, or tips. You could create one product that includes all items and then create shorter products for the individual items.

KEEPING ATTENTION: ENGAGEMENT

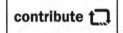 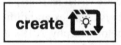

Add value to your content by engaging others in your work. Remember that social media is a way to build relationships within your network. If you are only putting content out but not engaging with your followers, that one-sided relationship isn't likely to be as fulfilling. It's not necessary to make every post engaging—in fact, that could be annoying—but think strategically about the best times and topics you use to do so. The following tips will help get your wheels turning on developing your engagement skills.

Engagement 101

When you create a post as a statement, it doesn't give your followers anything to respond to. If you want to know what your followers are thinking, engage with them.

Ask Open-Ended Questions

Transfer a basic principle of therapeutic communication into social media and this small tweak gives your followers something to respond to rather than just reading and scrolling on by your post. Ask for opinions, thoughts, feedback, recommendations; there's no limit as to what type of questions you can ask. For our qualitative researchers out there, this is one way to create an online focus group that you can analyze for themes!

Conduct a Poll

For our quantitative researcher friends, you may prefer to see statistics using a simple multiple-choice poll to engage your followers. In Twitter, you can have two to four poll answers; in Instagram, you add interactive stickers with two options that you drag-and-drop on a visual image; and Facebook has two poll options similar to Instagram but you can also use third-party apps to embed a poll on a Facebook Page (Nelson, 2018).

Check Back In

If you create a poll or ask a question, be sure that you check back in to follow up. Set a time limit and establish it within your poll or question. For example, "One Day Poll" and check in 24 hours after posting to follow up and close out the engagement.

Ask for or Make a Recommendation

In today's world, social media is where many people will look to find recommendations on products, services, and organizations. When we find something we love and/or makes our lives easier, sharing this via social media is another way to engage your audience.

Create a Hangout

You can do this by creating a private Facebook Group for a book club, support group, or information sharing. Again, the point here isn't to make the recommendation and leave the scene, but to engage with your audience in some type of experience or create a moment.

Create an Online Event

You can schedule a Facebook Live session where you share content on a certain topic or host a Facebook Watch Party. Introduced in 2018, a Facebook Watch Party is a way for people to watch live or recorded videos on Facebook and interact around them at the same time (Connolly, 2018).

Respond to Current Events With Your Unique Perspective

Every day, something new is going on in the world. Using social media and/or other outlets allows you to make a comment and offer your unique perspective on any given event, while building your brand and establishing yourself as an expert in your field.

A Unique Perspective

As the COVID pandemic was getting underway in mid-March of 2020, all major news outlets were reporting that older adults were at the highest risk for adverse illness resulting in increased risk for hospitalization and death. Older adults also do not typically present clinically with a fever for any infectious disease, but most media outlets were not reporting on the atypical presentation of illness in older adults. Using a podcast, blog, and social media format allowed adding to the mainstream conversation on atypical presentation of illness and ways to communicate with older relatives (Batchelor, 2020a, 2020b, 2020d).

Media Begets Media

In the previous example, the original video post led to traditional media engagements with a newspaper journalist (CNBC MakeIt) and two other radio interviews with NPR Weekend Edition Saturday and HealthCetera (Mason, 2020; Simon, 2020; Stieg, 2020).

Social Media Allows Others to Find You

And for this same example, the NPR interview resulted in another organization using social media (LinkedIn) to extend another invitation to speak at Nasdaq's Employee Assistance Program (Nasdaq, 2020). This cascade was truly a gift that kept on giving!

Testimonials

As people give you positive feedback, with their permission, you can post testimonials on your website to share this with your audience. Requesting a high-resolution photo or headshot of the person giving you the feedback that could accompany the quote is a way to ensure the authenticity of the comments, and also highlights and gives attention to your fans/audience/followers in a unique way.

Using Review Feedback

Whenever you get a compliment on your work, use it! Ask the person to write it up and for permission to post it. LinkedIn has a feature that allows for recommendations of your areas of expertise. Also, post patient testimonials or reviews for your organization or practice to help you attract new patients or employees.

Track Requests to Use Your Content

If someone contacts you and requests to use your content, keep a record of it. This demonstrates the impact of your work and can be a qualitative addition to your metrics. For example, if someone asks to include one of your videos in a related training program, it is a sign that your work is making a difference.

Throw It Back (or Two-Fer)

If you have created content in the past that is relevant to the current conversation, you can create your own "Throwback Thursday" (or something for other days of the week) where you retweet/reshare this content, updating it to apply to the current conversation. If you have written a blog, produced a video, published an article or any other "product" and it is the topic of conversation at a conference or in mainstream media, you can always use your archived product(s) and tag the current speaker, the conference, or the media outlet. Recycling relevant content is an opportunity to share that content with a new audience and potentially gain more followers in the process.

Use Email as a Constant Connector

Social media platforms will change over time, so putting all of your "eggs" into one basket is not an ideal strategy for staying connected with your target audience. Email will allow you to remain connected to your target audience even if Twitter or Facebook goes away—and allows you to email your followers any new platforms you may use as they pop up. To create your own professional email listserv, you can use an email platform like Mail Chimp, Mailer Lite, or any other program to help you manage the email addresses.

Building Your Email List

When you do presentations, you share information on how to subscribe to your email list to share news and events.

Email Best Practices

Some other examples are creating weekly videos or blogs with tips or whatever content fits your brand and area of expertise, and to send those out.

- If you're going to go through the effort to develop an email list, at the very least, send an email out at least a few times every year.
- If you are producing weekly content, you could email a "Monthly Round Up" every month. This allows anyone in your target audience who may not be on social media to see the weekly content in one place. You can also use email to announce new resources, news, or events that fit your brand and area of expertise.

- As with everything, put your most important content or message up front and chunk your content into scannable sections with bold headings. This allows a reader to quickly scan and understand your core message(s) and then decide which sections they will read and in what order.
- When possible, include a call to action, images, and/or links in your email. If you want your readers to do something, make it clear and easy to take action.

Email Analytics

The listserv you choose to use should also have some analytic ability to help you understand how your emails are performing. Normal non–work-related email open rates should be between 15% to 25% for an effective email campaign; average click-through rate around 2.5%; and your average click-to-open rate should be between 20% to 30% (Campaign Monitor, 2020). You can typically access these metrics through the Report feature with the email service provider used. These metrics can help you see which layout, links, copy, and overall content are most interesting to those on your email list as you try different email types, such as your welcome email, newsletter, or any campaigns you may launch to advertise products and services.

- **Email Open Rate.** This measure tells you how many email recipients open an email compared to the total number of emails sent.
- **Email Click-Through Rate.** This measure tells you how many of your email subscribers opened the email and clicked on a link within the body of the email.
- **Click-to-Open Rate.** This measure tells you the overall effectiveness of your email campaign and is calculated by the number of unique clicks divided by the number of unique opens.

Use Your Analytics

When you are starting out, be adventurous! Try creating different content products or topics and see how they play out with your followers. When you have one small success, use it to leverage future products you create. Over time, your followers will like and share your content with their followers—once something is out there, it can continue to gain momentum so don't lose hope if it's not an overnight success!

REFERENCES

@smfrogers. (2014, March 10). *What feuls a tweet's engagement?* blog.twitter.com. https://bit.ly/3as1NKb

Alzheimer's Impact Movement [@ALZIMPACT]. (2020, December 11). Negotiations on FY21 Appropriations packages continue as Congress is against another funding deadline. Join us in urging your members to [Image attached] [Tweet]. Twitter. https://bit.ly/3aujsRi

Animoto. (2020). *Choose a template teaser.* animoto.com. https://bit.ly/38hW46M

Apple Inc. (2020). *Apple Teacher.* https://apple.co/37CIHyW

Aurbach, E. L., Prater, K. E., Patterson, B., & Zikmund-Fisher, B. J. (2018). Half-life your message: A quick, flexible tool for message discovery. *Science Communication, 40*(5), 669-677. https://doi.org/10.1177/1075547018781917

Batchelor, M. [M. Batchelor]. (2017, March 2). Great resources from an Area Agency on Aging (AAA) - check one out the AAA in your community! via Ripl.com [Video attached] [Original post]. Facebook. https://bit.ly/38mWVDm

Batchelor, M. [@MelissaBPhD]. (2019a, October 2). Great work @MonaShattell & @BecDarmoc [Fisted hand emoji] Two in one week - next stop #Vegasbaby #socialmedia #GAPNA19 #Twitter [Image attached] [Retweet with comment]. [@MonaShattell]. Twitter. https://bit.ly/3nO8mKE

Batchelor, M. (2019b, October 19). *How a bill becomes a law.* YouTube [MelissaBPhD]. https://bit.ly/2KoIw1z

Batchelor, M. [@MelissaBPhD]. (2019c, September 25). Tip #1 to #AgeWell - Stand Up! #sitting is the new #smoking, so #GetUp and #MoveNaturally #AgeFriendly communities gave walkable spaces [Image attached] [Tweet]. Twitter. https://bit.ly/2KqjjDP

Batchelor, M. (Host). (2020a, March 23). Coronavirus and Older Adults (Episode 5) [Audiovisual podcast]. In: *This Is Getting Old: Moving Towards an Age-Friendly World.* https://bit.ly/3pbkbem

Batchelor, M. (Host). (2020b, June 1). Having the COVID conversation with older relatives (Episode 14) [Audiovisual podcast]. In: *This Is Getting Old: Moving Towards an Age-Friendly World.* https://bit.ly/34AW7tt

Batchelor, M. (Host). (2020c, July 14). How is alzheimer's diagnosed (Episode 19) [Audiovisual podcast]. In: *This Is Getting Old: Moving Towards an Age-Friendly World.* https://bit.ly/2WvagUL

Batchelor, M. (Host). (2020d, May 25). Recognizing risk factors & symptoms of COVID in older adults (Episode 13) [Audiovisual podcast]. In: *This Is Getting Old: Moving Towards an Age-Friendly World.* https://bit.ly/34vcQOH

Batchelor, M. (Host). (2020e, July 6). Six tips for talking to someone you think has a memory problem (Epsidoe 18) [Audiovisual podcast]. In: *This Is Getting Old: Moving Towards an Age-Friendly World.* https://bit.ly/2KFi3wC

Batchelor, M. (Host). (2020f, June 24). Ten signs of alzheimer's disease (Episode 17) [Audiovisual podcast]. In: *This Is Getting Old: Moving Towards an Age-Friendly World.* https://bit.ly/2WAQTcE

Batchelor-Murphy, M. (2019, August 6). *2018 update of the handfeeding demonstration video.* MelissaBPhD.com/NOSH. https://MelissaBPhD.com/NOSH

Bitable. (2020). *55 video marketing statistics for 2020.* https://bit.ly/3mAKDwd

BOLD Infrastructure for Alzheimer's Act, Pub. L. No. 115-406, S.2076/ H.R.4256 115th Cong. (2018). https://bit.ly/3mvdqCs

Campaign Monitor. (2020, November 20). *What are the average click and read rates for email campaigns?* The Marketing Resources Hub. https://bit.ly/38ZdjvF

Canva Pty Ltd. (2020). Canva: Graphic Design and Video (Version 3.84.0) [Mobile App]. App Store. https://apple.co/37ziuBj

Carr, N. (2020). *The shallows: what the internet is doing to our brains.* W. W. Norton & Company, Inc.

COMPASS Science Communications Inc. (2017). *The message box workbook: Communicating your science effectively.* https://bit.ly/2KqtoR8

Connolly, E. (2018, July 25). *Watch Party launches around the world.* about.facebook.com. https://bit.ly/2WDFatS

Darmoc, R. [@BecDarmoc]. (2020, July 30). Heading to meet up with @MonaShattell & @MelissaBPhD for our book writing weekend retreat! #maskup [Image attached] [Tweet]. Twitter. https://bit.ly/3nEOroF

Holidays Calendars. (n.d.). *Weird holiday calendars.* holidayscalendar.com. https://bit.ly/37zm5zG

Mansfield, M. (2020, December 26). *27 videos marketing statistics that will have you hitting the record button.* Small Business Trends. https://bit.ly/38oT1Lq

Mason, D. (2020, April 22). *COVID19 and older adults in nursing homes.* Healthcetera.

Nasdaq. (2020, May 7). *How to talk to your older relatives about the COVID-19 pandemic – and actually have them listen!.* Nasdaq Employee Assistance Program.

Nelson, N. (2018, July 8). *The power of social media polls: The drill-down on 3 platforms + 5 general best practices*. Top Rank Marketing. https://bit.ly/38qN1kg

O'Neill, M. (2020, January 31). *How long should videos be? FB, IG, YT & More in 2020*. Animoto. https://bit.ly/3rhx6NK

Oringe. (2020). WordSwag (Version 4.02.01) [Mobile app]. App Store. https://apple.co/3muXUGI

Ripl Inc. (2020). Ripl: Video and social posts (4.0.58) [Mobile app]. https://apple.co/3rkHPqw

Salshutz, E. (2017). *How to add captions to videos on Facebook*. Animoto.com. https://bit.ly/2Jd7AYS

Sellas, B. (2020, February 8). *10 ways to incorporate micro content into your social media strategy*. agorapulse.com. https://bit.ly/3rjnC4E

Simon, S. (Host). (2020, March 21). Don't Make them Feel Like a Charity Project: Talking to the Elderly About Coronavirus [Audio]. In: *NPR Weekend Edition Saturday*. https://n.pr/33NYxmR

Stieg, C. (2020, March 13). *How to talk with your older parents about the COVID-19 pandemic – and have them actually listen*. CNBC Make It. https://cnb.cx/2Uj5xoP

Tamble, M. (2019, February 20). *7 tips for using visual content marketing*. SocialMediaToday. https://bit.ly/38oOFny

Tech Insider. (2018, November 1). *How to record your iPhone screen*. YouTube. https://bit.ly/3mzNCVD

Templeman, M. (2017, September 6). *17 stats and facts every marketer should know about video marketing*. Forbes. https://bit.ly/39hkWvY

Unsplash Inc. (2020). Unsplash (Version 1.11.1) [Mobile app]. App Store. https://apple.co/34usvoY

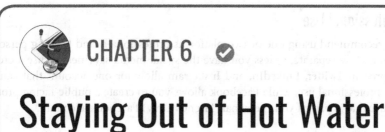

CHAPTER 6

Staying Out of Hot Water

👍 Like   ↪ Share

♡

"If you say things of consequence, there may be consequences.
The alternative is to be inconsequential."

Katie Orenstein
@katieorenst
@TheOpEdProject

PERSONAL OR PROFESSIONAL— HOW TO KNOW?

Boundaries Defined

What are the boundaries between professional and personal use of social media? We often get asked about whether you should have separate personal and professional accounts or personas. We tend to use one platform for more personal aspects of our lives (e.g., Facebook) and another for more professional purposes (e.g., Twitter and LinkedIn). We recommend that you are clear as to whether your account is professional or personal in your bio and make sure your privacy settings are set appropriately.

Shattell, M., Batchelor, M., & Darmoc, R. *Social Media in Health Care:*
A Guide to Creating Your Professional Digital Presence (pp. 91–100).
© 2022 Taylor & Francis Group.

Professional Use

We recommend using one or two platforms professionally and keeping personal posts completely separate, unless you have the social media savviness to use a cross-over approach. Twitter, LinkedIn, and Instagram allow for one account that can be used for professional use, while Facebook allows you to create a public-facing professional page that is part of your personal (Friends Only) Facebook account.

Personal Use

Social media for personal use includes sharing images or posts of your activities, family, and friends. On a personal account, you may share more religious or political views that may not be appropriate in a professional context. Remember to keep your personal posts clean enough to not impact you professionally. While sharing your professional work in your personal platform is likely going to be okay, sharing your personal life may not go so well on a platform you use professionally.

Crossover Use

You may choose to use a platform for professional and personal posts. One might use Facebook for posts about fun and family events, but use Twitter to post about the research findings from their latest study or about new practice guidelines that were just published. For example, we post professional content like op-eds that we author on our personal Facebook pages, and sometimes more personal posts on our Twitter accounts. We think this, if done well, provides for a more accurate and authentic representation. If you choose the crossover option, just be aware that any post can result in workplace ramifications.

BASIC RULES FOR ENGAGEMENT

Health care professionals maintain professional boundaries, know the policies of their organization, refrain from establishing duties of care through social media, protect their professional reputation, and create value-added posts. Health care professionals must comply with all applicable federal, state, and local laws and regulations relating to the privacy of patient health information put forth according to the Health Insurance Portability and Accountability Act (HIPAA) of 1996 ("Standards for privacy of individually identifiable health information. Final rule," 2000; "Standards for privacy of individually identifiable health information. Final rule," 2002).

And it's not just health care professionals that need to be concerned and careful. There have been many non–health care professionals who have learned that postings on social media can have a negative impact on one's career and activities, and we—those of us in the health care industry—can learn from them. We need to be aware that what we say on social media can have an impact on our jobs and careers.

As professionals, you want to Contribute positively to the social media realm and do not want to be fired or reprimanded, so you will want to follow patient privacy guidelines and any other published rules set by your workplace.

But What About Free Speech?

There is free speech, but free speech does not mean that we can break federal law or hospital or health system policies, and we must be concerned about our reputations. Remember that anything you put in writing—including tweets, images, and emails—can be shared widely. It is important now more than ever to be clear in your written messages and to know that technology and social media allows for easy dissemination, which is both the positive power and the potential pitfall.

Sharing and creating content on social media is a social activity—it's meant to be used by others, engaged with, and shared. Before you get started, or if you already are an active social media user, it's important to be aware of some potential pitfalls.

Social Media Meets HIPAA

As health care professionals who are responsible for the care of members of the community, who are privy to personal information, we must be sure to abide by privacy and confidentiality regulations, and social media is no exception. We are still bound by ethical standards that require us to protect patient privacy and keep patient information secure and confidential.

Another thing to keep in mind is that everything we type, post, share, text, or blog is discoverable. Patient information cannot be posted online in any social media platform. While this may be obvious, in today's world of easily sharable content, we must stop to think before we create a post. And remember, patient identifiable information is not just a person's name—it also includes any description or image.

According to Adler (2018), the most common HIPAA violations on social media are as follows: posting gossip about patients; posting of any information that identifies an individual; postings of images and videos of patients, family, or employees taken inside a health care facility without written consent; and sharing any patient health information (e.g., date of birth, Social Security numbers) on social media platforms or within any form of "private" online group.

WARNING: Hot Water for Professionals

There have been several instances when health care professionals posted identifiable patient information on social media and then were terminated. This was because their social media posts violated federal law, hospital policy, or both. There was the Texas nurse who was fired after posting a description on an anti-vaccination site about a child in their health care facility who tested positive for measles as reported in the *HIPAA Journal* (2018). Another example is a Navy corpsman (emergency medical technician) who was removed from their position after posting images of sick neonates (Eustachewich, 2017).

WARNING: Hot Water for Health Care Students

There was the first-year resident at AdventHealth in Orlando, Florida, Dr. Jay Feldman (@DrJayFeldman), who was reprimanded by their employer for the following post on Instagram:

"This one is for all the male medical students and residents that have been told to leave for the pelvic exam, who have been ignored during your OB/GYN rotation while the girls get to do all the learning. No more!!! Walk into that room with confidence! Show interest to your attending. You may never get another chance to learn this critical part of medicine! Don't blow it. Stand up for yourself" (Miller, 2019). This post was one among many that his employer received complaints about. The post was interpreted to mean female patients should be be allowed to refuse a male provider; an opinion the health system did not share

In addition to this post, Feldman also got into trouble for endorsing products—supplements used in raves and electronical dance music festivals—through his Instagram posts (Miller, 2019). This is problematic because as a doctor of osteopathy and family medicine resident, his views did not represent those of AdventHealth.

Lack of Social Media Training. Sarah Mojared (@Sarah_Mojarad) calls the endorsing of products "White Coat Marketing" and thinks it's a bad thing for physicians to do. There is little training that physicians, nurses, and other health care professionals get on what they can and should not do on social media. In the words of Feldman:

"No one ever teaches you how to do these things. There was never any formal training and so you just kind of figure it out as you go along. It makes a lot of sense that I shouldn't be using my medical degree as a platform to sell products. But no one teaches you this stuff" (Miller, 2019).

But What About Academic Freedom?

The term "academic freedom" typically applies for those of us who are in education. You might remember years earlier, professor Steven Salaita who had his job offer at the University of Illinois rescinded because the university did not agree with his tweets about Israel and the ongoing conflict with Hamas (Alexander & Alexander, 2015). In this case, Salaita sued the university and won, but has not been able to secure a long-term academic post, and now apparently drives a school bus in the suburbs of Washington, DC (Pettit, 2019).

WARNING: Hot Water for Faculty

You don't want to be the White criminology professor at the University of North Carolina Wilmington who wrote inflammatory posts during the COVID pandemic about the slow re-opening of the state of North Carolina: "This evening I ate pizza and drank beer with six guys at a six seat [sic] table top. I almost felt like a free man who was not living in the slave state of North Carolina. Massa Cooper, let my people go!" And another post that he wrote: "Don't shut down the universities. Shut down the non-essential [sic] majors. Like Women's Studies" (Alfonso, 2020). The university investigated the controversial social media posts, many of which were viewed as racist, sexist, or homophobic in nature. The faculty member sued the university and received a $500,000 settlement after agreeing to retire (WTVD-AP, 2020); he was protected by free speech in the First Amendment as his tweets were his opinions and not related to his work as a university professor (Baird, 2014).

Using Your Powers for Good

There are so many examples of people who lost positions, jobs, roles, or reputation because of words that they wrote on social media or video or audio that was captured and shared. And what might go unnoticed in one historical context, is flammable and not tolerated in another.

WARNING: Public Dialogue

During the #JusticeForGeorgeFloyd protests against #RacismInAmerica, several individuals who posted or said racist words were immediately terminated from their jobs.

WARNING: Business Leaders

The CEO of Crossfit Greg Glassman "retired" (or resigned) after making racist statements about #GeorgeFloyd and the #BlackLivesMatter movement (Gorman & Taylor, 2020).

WARNING: Authors

J.K. Rowling, author of the Harry Potter series, received wide criticism for her anti-trans tweets and follow-up explanations (Kelly, 2020).

WARNING: Athletes

New Orleans Saints quarterback Drew Brees made an unsupportive comment about the Colin Kaepernick #TakeaKnee campaign, which was a silent protest against police brutality and the murder of Black men. Brees said it was disrespectful of the flag (Brees eventually apologized; Belson, 2020).

This is not meant to scare you away from engaging with social media but instead to remind you of potential pitfalls. Now let's talk about several resources that can help guide your social media practice as a health care professional.

Resources to Stay Out of Hot Water

There are several toolkits and online resources from health care organizations that help guide health care professionals—on ways to avoid pitfalls, share health information, and promote the health professions.

Questions to Ask Yourself

- Is your post positive?
- Is your post informative?
- Is your post factual?
- Does your post engage readers?
- Does this post enhance or detract from your professional reputation?
- Does this post break any laws or breach any ethical standards?

Journals

The *HIPAA Journal* published a guide to "HIPAA and Social Media" since the original HIPAA came into being before social media was as ubiquitous as it is today (*HIPAA Journal*, 2018).

National Professional Organizations

There are a variety of resources to keep you out of hot water as health care professionals using social media.

- American Nurses Association Social Media (available online for free), or can be purchased as an eBook for $4.95 (American Nurses Association, 2011)
- The American Hospital Association (American Hospital Association & Society for Healthcare Strategy & Market Development, 2015)

Government Agencies

- CDC's Guide to Writing for Social Media (Center for Disease Control and Prevention, 2012)
- CDC, The Health Communicator's Social Media Toolkit (Centers for Disease Control and Prevention, 2011)

Your Workplace Social Media Policy

If you are employed by a health care organization, university, or other company, we encourage you to find and read their social media policy. You might also review any policy related to behavior. For those who want to use images of patients in educational or marketing materials, you will need to review your organization's policies on gaining patient consent.

Declare That Views and Opinions Are Your Own in Your Bio

When we talk about social media and public thought leadership, our views are put out into the world and we must be prepared for what can happen. You are entitled to free speech to share your opinions and to "be political" by voicing your political views. However, what you say has the potential to touch a nerve with some who have a different opinion or an opposing view. Be prepared for someone who doesn't like what you say on social media; you may have to deal with some backlash.

Backlash From Haters and Trolls

Digital and virtual formats make it easy for "haters" and "trolls" to drop in.

What Is a Hater?

The meaning of a hater is a person who doesn't like what you have to say and is confrontational about their opposing views.

What Is a Troll?

The meaning of troll—a troll, to troll—has evolved over time. A "troll" as a noun is used to refer to a mythical ugly creature. As a verb, "to troll" was to drop a fishing line in the water off the side of a boat and then pick up whatever you can while the boat is moving through the water. In social media, a troll is a person who maliciously looks for people to aggravate, push their buttons, and disagree in an antagonistic, hurtful, and acerbic way. "Trolls typically latch onto 'hot-button issues' with emotional resonance: Gun control, immigration ... They make outrageous, inflammatory comments in the hopes that you'll lose your cool" (Shaffer, 2016). Remember that their sole intention is to hurt and to silence.

If this has not happened to you yet, it likely will, so you should be prepared. Sharing the fact that you will have haters and trolls should not scare or silence you. For anyone using social media professionally, it's good for you to consider ahead of time how you will react and respond when someone is mean and nasty to your knowledge and ideas.

Scenario: The Tweet

As an example, a tweet posted that reflected on use of the title "Dr." read, "The more I think about it, #PhD #DNP & other term degrees NEED to fully reclaim 'Dr.' PhDs were called 'Dr' before MDs were ..." (Shattell, 2017).

A couple of followers took offense and disagreed with the tweet.

Hater Response

One follower replied, "DNP is not equivalent to MD/DO. It is typically an online degree obtained to trick pts into thinking the provider is a medical doctor. The training is a fraction of that of a medical doctor yet DNP seek parity with them. It's a scam" (MAGADOC, 2018).

Troll Response

"'Doctorly-Prepared Nurses'—are doing nothing to improve access to care, they're opening dangerous unsupervised cosmetic clinics and they are worsening the bedside RN shortage—which is an actual shortage—and much worse than the so-called 'physician shortage'" (ConcernedMD, 2018).

In any scenario like this, you have to decide what to do, if anything. Here are some ideas for how to manage negative comments.

Tips for Managing Haters and Trolls

Don't Take It Personally

Health care professionals are accustomed to being evaluated in clinical or academic settings. Academics are used to being evaluated by peers and students alike. There are patient satisfaction surveys, student and course evaluations, the peer review process for submitted academic manuscripts, and annual and mid-year reviews for faculty members and administrators. Just like these types of performance evaluations should not be taken personally, neither should responses to your social media posts.

Distinguish Haters From Well-Meaning Critics

Decide if other people's comments on your posts are constructive or destructive. You will get positive and negative feedback, just try not to focus on the negative. As you would do with any feedback, you must decide if there is truth to the critique or anything you can do to improve.

Correct Misinformation

Take this opportunity to correct misinformation from the comments. Difference of opinion is fine, but misinformation is not. In this scenario, it did not appear that these responders were interested in knowing the real data, real research about NP practice or about the RN shortage or the primary care provider shortage. It didn't appear that the responders were interested in a dialogue or debate about the issues.

Take It Offline

If you want to have a longer conversation with someone where there might be an opportunity to understand each other better, or you want to address bad behavior in a private setting, use direct messaging to contact the person with a private message.

Block or Mute

In Twitter, use the Mute and Block features. Do not engage with the hater or troll. Simply ignore them and forget about it, but don't let it silence you.

Report Abuse

For especially aggressive behavior, you can also report accounts who are abusive, threatening, harassing, or "direct hate against a protected category (e.g., race, religion, gender, orientation, disability)" (Twitter Help Center, n.d.).

Scenario: Resolution

In this scenario, we only shared the initial tweet and first responses by a hater and a troll, but the conversation continued among other tweeters. The hater disengaged from the dialogue, but the troll became increasingly belligerent with their posts.

While others engaged with the troll, the decision by the original tweet poster was to ignore it and move on. As the troll continued to post, they were blocked and muted so the initial tweeter wasn't bothered anymore, but the conversation continued.

At the end of the day:

"The less you respond to negative people, the more peaceful your life will become."

Unknown

REFERENCES

Adler, S. (2018, March 12). *HIPAA social media rules*. HIPPA Journal. https://bit.ly/3mJqpQU

Alexander, H., & Alexander, N. (2015, January 29). *Anti-Isreal professor sues university of Illinois for re-scinding job offer*. Haaretz. https://bit.ly/3h2g7u1

Alfonso, F. (2020, June 7). *University of North Carolina Wilmington calls professor's tweets 'vile and inex-cusable' following growing backlash online*. https://cnn.it/3r7NVKW

American Hospital Association, & Society for Healthcare Strategy & Market Development. (2015, May). *A hospital leadership guide to digital and social media engagement*. American Hospital Association. https://bit.ly/395dTGN

American Nurses Association. (2011). *Social media*. American Nurses Association. https://bit.ly/3p8aRbb

Baird, P. (2014, March 20). *Professor wins lawsuit against UNCW*. StarNews Online. https://bit.ly/3i8IcRE

Belson, K. (2020, June 4). *Drew Brees' unchanged stance on kneeling is suddenly out of step*. New York Times. https://nyti.ms/3nGDuvG

Centers for Disease Control and Prevention. (2011). *The health communicator's social media toolkit*. Office of the Associate Director for Communication. https://www.cdc.gov/healthcommunication/ToolsTemplates/SocialMediaToolkit_BM.pdf

Centers for Disease Control and Prevention. (2012, April). *CDC's guide to writing social media*. Electronic Media Branch, Division of News and Electronic Media, Office of the Associate Director for Communication,. https://bit.ly/34sPOIC

ConcernedMD [@MdConcerned]. (2018, December 8). "Doctorly-Prepared Nurses" - are doing noth-ing to improve access to care, they're opening dangerous unsupervised cosmetic clinics and they are [Comment]. @MonaShattell. Twitter. https://bit.ly/3pFuSG8

Eustachewich, L. (2017, September 19). *Naval staffers booted over disturbing pics, posts of 'mini-satan' newborns*. New York Post. https://bit.ly/38nGbMa

Gorman, A., & Taylor, J. (2020, June 10). *CrossFit CEO resigns after offensive George Floyd and coronavirus tweets*. The Guardian. https://bit.ly/3rmOIHR

HIPAA Journal. (2018, March 12). *HIPPA social media rules*. HIPAA Journal. https://bit.ly/3anRTcx

HIPPA Journal. (2018, September 13). *Texas nurse fired for social media HIPAA violation*. HIPPA Journal. https://bit.ly/38iLNHD

Kelly, S. (2020, June 7). *'Harry Potter' author J.K. Rowling's tweets blasted for being anti-transgender*. Los Angeles Times. https://lat.ms/37J4Vj7

MAGADOC [@ERPatriot]. (2018, December 13). DNP is not equivalent to MD/DO. It is typically an online degree obtained to trick pts into thinking the [Comment]. @MonaShattell. Twitter. https://bit.ly/3pDbSbw

Miller, N. (2019, December 14). *AdventHealth resident in hot water for social media posts, side-gig*. Orlando Sentinel. https://bit.ly/2KzyHho

Pettit, E. (2019, February 19). *'Ousted' from academe, Steven Salaita says he's driving a school bus to make ends meet*. The Chronicle of Higher Education. https://bit.ly/3iDQa5Q

Shaffer, A. (2016, July 12). *You can't plan for internet hate, but you can be prepared for it*. Inc.com. https://bit.ly/3niJMkc

Shattell, M. [@MonaShattell]. (2017, May 27). the more I think about it, #PhD #DNP & other term degrees NEED to fully reclaim "Dr". PhDs were called [Tweet]. Twitter. https://bit.ly/2JLTPAI

Standards for privacy of individually identifiable health information. Final rule, 45 CFR 160 45 CFR 164 Department of Health and Human Services, Office of the Assistant Secretary for Planning and Evaluation, Federal Register. (2000). https://bit.ly/2Xf8Xtc

Standards for privacy of individually identifiable health information. Final rule., 45 CFR 160 45 CFR 164 Department of Health and Human Services, Office of the Secretary, Federal Register. (2002). https://bit.ly/2JIUpz6

Twitter Help Center. (n.d.). *Report a violation*. Twitter. https://bit.ly/2XmjJhm

WTVD-AP. (2020, July 3). *UNC Wilmington professor gets 500K settlement and backlash over racist social media comments*. ABC 11 TV. https://abc11.tv/3asWudk

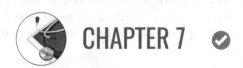

CHAPTER 7 ✅

Blending Gold Standards and Innovation in Sharing Knowledge and Expertise

👍 Like   ↪ Share

♡   💬   ⇄

"The trailblazers in human, academic, scientific and religious freedom have always been nonconformists."

Martin Luther King Jr.

WHY SHOULD YOU BLEND TRADITIONAL AND MODERN DISSEMINATION STRATEGIES?

Publish or Perish

As a health care professional or academic, or in your role as a leader in your organization or profession, publishing is a cornerstone of sharing traditional scientific findings. The primary purpose of traditional scholarly dissemination is to clearly communicate your ideas and findings to a broader scientific community. Communicating in writing—clearly and succinctly—is a skill needed by students and professionals alike. This form of peer-reviewed communication has been, and will continue to be, the gold standard for establishing your

Shattell, M., Batchelor, M., & Darmoc, R. *Social Media in Health Care: A Guide to Creating Your Professional Digital Presence* (pp. 101-112).

expertise, but the time has come to take our scholarship to the next level. This modality of communication results in a 17-year timeline for science to be integrated into evidence-based practice and public consumption—but there is a way to shorten this interval.

But in Today's World, It Is Not Enough

Use of social media sites in the past decade has increased exponentially, and can be used as an alternate form of communicating health information. In 2021, 72% of Americans reported using social media networking sites (Auxier & Anderson, 2021). Social media has changed the way many people get information and how they share it in their daily lives with some differences demographically. While the majority of social media users are younger adults (18 to 29 [84%]; 30 to 49 [81%]), older adults are also getting in the game (50 to 64 [73%]; 65 and older [45%]; Auxier & Anderson, 2021).

How the Public Accesses Health Information

When accessing online health information, using Google or another search engine is the primary way both older adults (37%) and family and friends (61%) go about it, but both groups have varying levels of confidence in their ability to find reliable, accurate, and/or trustworthy information (Turner et al., 2018). Using MedlinePlus, nonprofit national association websites (e.g., AARP), or a patient portal to access online health information were rarely reported as ways of accessing online health information (Turner et al., 2018).

Influence of Health Care Professionals

As a local health care professional, you are most frequently reported as the first and best source of health information for your patients (Turner et al., 2018). If your organization is creating content that directly helps your patient population, and identifies trusted resources, your patients will visit your website first to learn more about a given health topic. If you are online, your patients will have 24/7 access to information they will feel they can trust.

Personal Professional Website

Having a personal professional website is a way to manage your online presence. Some universities offer free hosting through WordPress for hosting faculty websites, or you may need to develop your own (UCI Faculty Websites, 2020). Other choices for website builders include Wix, Squarespace, Site 123, and HostGator. Many of these have plans and some level of pricing, so investigate the monthly or annual fees to find the pricing that fits your budget. It's best to match your domain name to your brand,

and your website builder can let you know if your choice is available. Having your own, independent website means that all your content goes with you if you decide to change employers. Your website can also function as a living résumé for you if designed to do so.

Generational Differences

While there is a notable digital divide between the generations of young and old, older adults do rely heavily on family and friends to seek and understand health information (Anderson & Perrin, 2017). Older adults trust health care professionals (85%) and family and friends (55%) as their primary sources for health information; and family and friends most often use the internet (54%) as their primary source of health information (Anderson & Perrin, 2017; Turner et al., 2018). Younger generations are much more likely to search YouTube and the internet to access health information. As a health care professional, you can translate complex medical information for your patient population in a way that is engaging and gets their attention. A peer-reviewed publication won't have the same mileage as a short video clip viewed more than 1000 times.

How Policymakers Find Experts

Google. Given the restrictions on access to peer-reviewed journal articles and the lack of skills to search institutional databases, a non-academic member of the public is most likely going to turn to the internet to find the answer to any question they may have. If you don't have a professional web presence, policymakers aren't going to be able to find you. By turning your peer-reviewed publications and professional presentations into a product consumable by the public, you are increasing your odds of being identified as an expert in your field and having your expertise sought after.

TRADITIONAL DISSEMINATION STRATEGIES

The "most widely accepted medium for formal scholarly communication continues to be the published article in a peer-reviewed, scientific journal" (American Psychological Association [APA], 2020). Researchers and scholars alike are taught that research is not complete until the findings or results of their work are shared through publication in a scientific journal (APA, 2020). These journal articles allow authors to make original contributions with appropriate citations to reference the work of others and serve as the repository of primary research literature accumulated to advance knowledge in a field of inquiry (APA, 2020).

Traditional Peer-Reviewed Publications

In academic health care programs, students are taught to write scholarly scientific papers using the publication manuals of the APA or the American Medical Association (American Medical Association, 2020; APA, 2020). This style of writing is formal and based on principles that students and professionals alike follow as the publication standards that encompass the legal, ethical, and professional principles (APA, 2020). The process of writing allows students and professionals to engage in scientific inquiry, critical thinking, and self-reflection (APA, 2020).

Scientific journals publish a variety of journal article types, including qualitative, quantitative, and mixed methods empirical articles (APA, 2020). Each type of manuscript has its own distinct sections and authors must consider the article topic and type to determine the appropriate journal to submit it to. The same holds true for using social media venues (Table 7-1).

Publication + Social Media

In today's world of publication, publishers are tapping into the power of using social media to promote books, journals, authors, and publications. When you submit a manuscript, you may be asked to provide your professional social media information for platforms such as Twitter and/or LinkedIn. You may be asked to draft a tweet the publisher can use when the article is released.

When submitting to a publication, be sure to find the publisher's social media connection across platforms. The hyperlinked icons for each platform can usually be found on the publisher's website. Follow publishers and any journals that you submit manuscripts to or that focus on an area of interest to you. It's highly likely that all traditional scholarship will be shared via social media, so this is another reason to have a professional online presence.

By liking and following journalists, publishers, colleagues, and other organizations, you can like/retweet content related to your area of research, scholarship, or clinical practice. Monitoring social media also allows you to celebrate the successes of your colleagues in a public forum (the 80-20 rule). When you see publications shared/mentioned that were written by colleagues, you can like/share/retweet the original post, tagging your organization, adding relevant hashtags, and tagging the author(s). Publishing is already challenging, and everyone loves cheers and acknowledgment of their publication endeavors. Your assistance promoting their work will likely be reciprocated and allows your work to spread farther than ever before.

Twitter in the Classroom

If you are a faculty member assigning reading from a textbook, include the author's social media information (if you know it). You can create a Twitter assignment in your course and have students find and follow 10 influencers in the area of scholarship relevant to the course and/or student interest. For example, in a health policy course,

TABLE 7-1. TIPS BY THE 3C'S

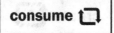

Traditional Publications

- Find the social media connections and follow publishers and any journals you submit manuscripts to.
- Like, share, retweet publications of colleagues on social media.
- Like, share, retweet your publication social media announcement from the publisher.
- Submit effective social media messaging to individual publishers for sharing your work via social media.
- Include author Twitter handles for assigned readings (in classroom).

Presentations

- Include your social media information on the first and last slide of any PowerPoint presentations with relevant hashtags in the slide footer.
- Based on conference format, include the most relevant social media handle in the slide footer.

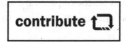

Traditional Publications

- Retweet your publication announcement on the journal's social media platform with a comment about why the publication is important.

Presentations

- Include your social media information (and that of your organization) at the beginning, end, and along the bottom of each slide.
- In presentations, include relevant hashtags for content in the body of the slide.
- Use an organizational template if it is available but if not, tailor the poster with colors, fonts, and logos you have developed for you and your professional brand.
- If you created your poster in PowerPoint, save it as a .jpg file and upload the image to your social media platforms.
- Take a photo of a slide during a presentation and post with comment.

(continued)

TABLE 7-1. TIPS BY THE 3C'S (CONTINUED)

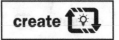

Traditional Publications

- Record a video (or audio) abstract for your publications, including your social media information.
  - Tweet your recorded video (or audio) abstract for your publications.
  - Add your recorded video (or audio) abstract from your publications to your professional website.

Presentations

- Create and schedule social media coverage (e.g., tweets) about your presentation to launch during your scheduled presentation time.
- Create and include a QR code on your poster to connect your audience directly to additional online content.

if you are using Dr. Diana Mason's textbook, for any assigned readings where she is an author, include @djmasonrn and encourage students to follow her.

Publication + Video

Using video is becoming increasingly popular as a powerful communication tool, but researchers and clinicians often overlook video as an option to promote written materials. Creating a video abstract of your publication allows you to engage with your audience through a short verbal communication. Adding a video to your social media post will increase your views by 48% (Bitable, 2020). A tweet with video increases retweeting an average of 28% (@smfrogers, 2014). In the business world, 59% of executives report preferring to watch a video over reading text. In short, many of us will watch a short video whereas we may not read a 500-word abstract (Bitable, 2020).

Create Your Own Video Abstract

Creating a video also allows you and your institution to share the publication announcement though a video abstract across multiple social media channels. You can use screenshots of social media posts and/or embed the video in conference presentations, share with the local press office, and include the link in future grant applications or other publications (Author Services, 2020a).

Core Message

Given that your goal is to have a short video, think about your core message. One strategy to help you focus and frame your video abstract is doing a process to Half-Life Your Message (Aurbach et al., 2018). In this process, you progressively compress your messaging from 60 seconds to 30 seconds to 15 seconds. This process will help you to determine your central message, key points you want to make, and the ideas/topics you need to present to support your central message (Aurbach et al., 2018). This process also helps with message prioritization—you only need to give enough information to intrigue a viewer into reading your abstract and article.

Scripting

Another way to create a video abstract is to draft a script. Keep in mind that your audience may not be as familiar with your work, so avoid jargon as much as possible. Given that many of us write much differently than we talk, you may find it helpful to sketch a short outline of the key message and two to three supporting statements and dictate your words into a program that will convert it to text for you. Scripting may also help prevent stumbling on using filler words (e.g., "um", "like"). Then when you read your script on video, you sound much more relaxed and natural than you would if you read your written statement.

Production

After you have created your video, it's worth developing a few basic skills with iMovie to create a thumbnail photo and edit out any errors. There are many resources available for free to assist you with this skill development—from the Apple Store Support (https://support.apple.com/imovie), YouTube tutorials, or becoming an Apple Teacher (https://appleteacher.apple.com). Apple Teacher provides succinct, self-paced modules to teach you how to use iMovie, Keynote, and GarageBand if you'd like to create your own music. If you don't want to get fancy or overly involved, just insert a single PowerPoint slide into a .jpg at the front of your video abstract, and this solves the thumbnail problem and can help you incorporate your brand into each video abstract.

Post-Production

Upload your video abstract to your YouTube Channel. From this point, you can embed it into your professional website (if you have one) or just share the link through social media posts. Another option would be to create a free QR code and insert the QR code into your poster or podium presentations.

Create a Video Abstract Through the Journal

Publishers may offer you the opportunity to record a short video abstract (3 to 5 minutes or less; Author Services, 2020a, 2020b; BMJ Author Hub, 2020). Taking the time to do this extra step can allow your peer-reviewed publication to engage with a broader audience, increase the visibility of your work (over 110% higher full text view), and improve your impact on article metrics (over 445% improved Altmetric score; Author Services, 2020a, 2020b).

Follow the Guidelines

Each publisher provides guidelines regarding length of the video, accessibility (provide written transcript for closed captioning), use of images (charts, tables, or figures included in the publication), and/or having a call to action (e.g., policy implications) (Author Services, 2020b). Be aware that some publishers will offer this service for free while others may charge $500 to $1750. We would recommend exploring the free options rather than paying out-of-pocket. However, when writing a grant or if your work is funded, this is a viable and innovative form of dissemination to include in your budget (if applicable).

Understand Video Copyrights

Be sure you understand the copyright terms of the video abstract—often they are the same copyright terms as the associated article (BMJ Author Hub, 2020). Work with individual journal publishers to understand the license (exclusive license and/or a non-exclusive license) for your publication and video so that you know how to best promote your work after the video abstract is released. If the work remains on the journal's website, you can embed the video in your own professional website to further promote the article and video. Be sure to hyperlink the video to the publication if you link or publish the video on your own website.

TRADITIONAL PRESENTATIONS

Presentations and posters are typically easier to do than get a manuscript published. That being said, traditional peer-reviewed publications are the highest ranked form of dissemination for academic settings. In fact, the adage in academics is that, "every poster should have a paper"; however, both forms of communication are highly valuable in sharing your work.

Poster and podium presentations are another traditional way to communicate research findings, clinical results, and/or educational strategies at professional conferences in a visual or oral manner (Zerwic et al., 2010). Both types of presentations require the presenter develop basic public speaking skills and can advance your science and build your professional network. Presenters must also consider how to present information in a visual way that attracts attention and engages conference participants.

Podium Presentations

Podium presentations are typically regarded as the best method for doing an oral presentation. This allows the presenter to reach a larger audience at one time and typically have a short Q&A time built in to allow audience participation.

Stay Connected + Weekly Podcast

Website: https://melissabphd.com/podcastblog/
YouTube: Melissa B PhD
Facebook: Melissa B PhD
LinkedIn: Melissa Batchelor
Twitter: @MelissaBPhD
Instagram: MelissaBPhD_thenurse

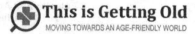

This is Getting Old
MOVING TOWARDS AN AGE-FRIENDLY WORLD

Podcast platforms:
Search "*Melissa B PhD This is Getting Old*"
- iTunes
- Spotify
- Stitcher

Figure 7-1. Slide with social media information.

Include Social Media

When preparing a podium presentation, you should integrate your brand and include your social media information at the beginning and end of your presentation and include your handle and relevant hashtags along the bottom of your slide (Figure 7-1). We include our Twitter handles and relevant, trending hashtags within the presentation (Figure 7-2). You can also include other social media platforms you use at the beginning and end of your presentation (e.g., LinkedIn, Instagram, YouTube Channel, website link) to all platforms you use professionally. This allows audience members to tweet/post while you are presenting, use your handle/name, use the recommended hashtags for your content, and follow you on platforms they are on. This is a great way to build your network and maintain contact with others long after your one-time presentation ends.

Be Creative

When preparing a podium presentation (PowerPoint, Keynote, Prezi), use an organizational template if it is available; if not, tailor the presentation with colors, fonts, and logos you have developed for you and your professional brand. For some presentations, we have told our story using only hashtags, handles, and graphics (Figure 7-3). This created a visually appealing presentation that engaged our audience and made it easier for those listening to promote our work using social media during the presentation.

Create Tip

Twitter will allow you to create and pre-schedule tweets to go out from you at a specified time during your presentation since you can't tweet and present at the same time. This allows your audience members to see your tweets and then retweet them.

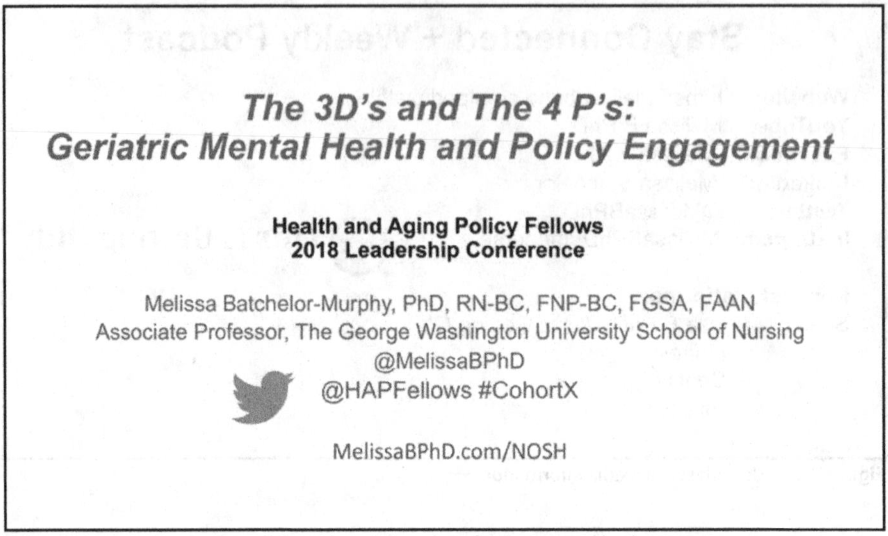

Figure 7-2. First presentation slide with social media information and hashtags.

Poster Presentations

Poster presentations allow for visual communication of your work with a smaller, one-to-one interaction with others who may drop by to check out your work.

Include Social Media

Include your social media contact information on your poster and if you recorded a video abstract for a paper you are presenting, include a QR code linked to the video abstract on poster presentations. When preparing a poster presentation, use an organizational template if it is available; if not, tailor the poster with colors, fonts, and logos you have developed for you and your professional brand. Be sure to include all your social media contact information (e.g., Twitter, Instagram, Facebook, LinkedIn, YouTube Channel) and that of your co-authors.

During Your Poster Presentation

You could do a (selfie) Facebook Live video sharing your poster during your conference poster presentation time, or ask a colleague to video-record your presentation interaction with a conference-goer (to post on other social media outlets afterward). If sharing through other social media sites, be sure to include the conference hashtag and your organization's handle and tag any co-authors or persons in the video with you. These strategies will help with cross-promotion between you, other conference-goers, and your organizational social media outlets.

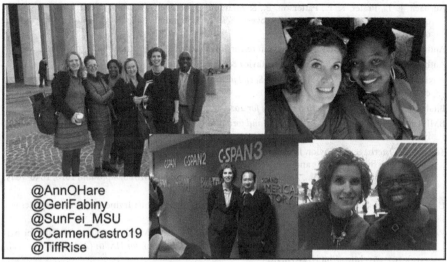

Figure 7-3. Slide with photos and handles.

Post Poster Presentation

After the live event, the conference may post the abstract online. If you created your poster in PowerPoint, save it as a .jpg file and upload the image to your social media platforms. Consider recording an audio abstract if you don't have any video footage. An easy way to do this is to upload the PowerPoint or .jpg version to Zoom and record a short presentation on your poster using the Zoom platform's Record feature. When you are done recording, the saved .mp4 file can be uploaded to your YouTube Channel to share across social media platforms, post to your website, or link to your faculty/professional bio within your organization or institution.

In tandem with the traditional dissemination of original research through peer-reviewed publication and presentations at scientific conferences, scholars need to have another layer to their communication strategy. These ideas are meant to help you do that within the 3C's Model of Social Media Development.

REFERENCES

@smfrogers. (2014, March 10). *What feuls a tweet's engagement?* blog.twitter.com. https://bit.ly/3as1NKb

American Medical Association. (2020). *AMA manual of style: A guide for authors and editors* (11th ed.). Oxford University Press. https://doi.org/10.1093/jama/9780190246556.001.0001

American Psychological Association. (2020). *Publication manual of the American Psychological Association* (7th ed.). https://doi.org/https://doi.org/10.1037/0000165-000

Anderson, M., & Perrin, A. (2017, May). *Tech adoption climbs among older adults.* Pew Research Center. https://www.pewresearch.org/internet/2017/05/17/technology-use-among-seniors/

Aurbach, E. L., Prater, K. E., Patterson, B., & Zikmund-Fisher, B. J. (2018). Half-life your message: A quick, flexible tool for message discovery. *Science Communication, 40*(5), 669-677. https://doi.org/10.1177/1075547018781917

Author Services. (2020a, May 13). *Share you research with videos.* Wiley. https://bit.ly/3nxUVyH

Author Services. (2020b). *Video abstracts.* Taylor & Francis. https://bit.ly/3h5cMKH

Auxier, B., & Anderson, M. (2021, April 7). *Social media use in 2021.* Pew Research Center. https://pewrsr.ch/3rHqSZe

Bitable. (2020). *55 video marketing statistics for 2020.* https://bit.ly/3mAKDwd

BMJ Author Hub. (2020, May 13). *Writing and formatting: Video abstracts.* BMJ Author Hub. https://bit.ly/2KhKrF7

Turner, A., Osterhage, K., Taylor, J., Hartzler, A., & Demiris, G. (2018). A closer look at health information seeking by older adults and involved family and friends: Design considerations for health information technologies. AMIA ... Annual Symposium proceedings. *AMIA Symposium, 2018*, 1036-1045. https://bit.ly/3nxUEf1

UCI Faculty Websites. (2020). *Faculty Web Page.* University of California Irvine. https://faculty.sites.uci.edu

Zerwic, J., Grandfield, K., Kavanaugh, K., Berger, B., Graham, L., & Mershon, M. (2010). Tips for better visual elements in posters and podium presentations. *Education for Health (Abingdon, England), 23*(2), 267-267. https://bit.ly/2KynDRf

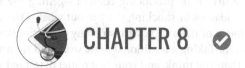

CHAPTER 8 ✅

Using Social Media to Engage Traditional Media

👍 **Like**   ↪ **Share**

♡   💬   ⇄

"Activism is something we are all responsible for. It is not something we turn over to a group of people. It's either in our daily lives or it's not."

Glennon Doyle
@GlennonDoyle

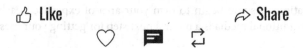

BEING AN ADVOCATE IS ALREADY IN YOUR DNA

As a health care professional, you advocate for many different things—from your patients to better population health outcomes to improvements in patient safety measures. You also most likely have other passions in the world of advocacy, but do you voice those opinions publicly? Your advocacy as a professional and as a human being can intersect through social media and be amplified through traditional media.

Stories Capture Attention

For social and traditional media, the news is all about trending issues in politics, health care, any consumer interest or concern, and pop culture. The news is

Shattell, M., Batchelor, M., & Darmoc, R. *Social Media in Health Care:*
A Guide to Creating Your Professional Digital Presence (pp. 113-121).
© 2022 Taylor & Francis Group.

about storytelling. News outlets are driven by producing content—getting the best, newest, and sometimes the most scandalous or shocking story about what is trending in the moment. Within these categories of news topics are so many opportunities for you to get involved in the conversation. Taking a traditional news story and framing it to fit your area of expertise is easier than you think, and your first outlet to test out your activism is on social media.

The 24-Hour News Cycle

Both social media and traditional media are working 24 hours a day, 7 days a week, 365 days a year. Traditional media needs stories and if they are related to health care, your voice is needed. Traditional media needs content to fill network airtime, print, and e-publications. As you begin to own your area of expertise, reaching further to engage with traditional media is a natural next step for getting your message out to the public.

We've all seen how the narrative in the news changes on a dime. A new scandal erases coverage of another scandal. Sometimes the topics are so monumental that the news covers it for weeks or months. We saw this happen with the COVID-19 pandemic. It happens during our cycle of political transitions and fighting between political parties. It happens when regular people rise up to declare and defend their rights through social movements and protests. No matter your news source, they are covering what is happening right now, in the moment.

You Can Achieve Things Much Larger Than Yourself

Policy, practice, research, and social movements affect public health. If not you, then who will do it? Using your voice to convey expert advice cuts through all the misinformation and conspiracy theories of the uninformed and unscientific public opinions that are crowding our digital sources of information. But you must want to be in the conversation. You must have passion for your viewpoints and causes. It's easy to say this is a given, considering you are a health care professional and your passion is to help others. We are just suggesting that you take it a step further than your clinical practice, research, or education responsibilities. You don't have to be gregarious or attention-seeking; you just have to be willing to put yourself out into the public in a new way, with your authentic brand guiding the way.

WHAT IS TRADITIONAL MEDIA?

Traditional media includes television, radio, newspapers, magazines, and the online versions of these outlets mirror the same content (e.g., FoxNews.com, CNN.com, NPR.org, NYTimes.com, WSJ.com, ScientificAmerican.com, ModernHealthcare.com).

Traditional media still runs on fixed rules of journalism that have been around for decades. As a profession, journalists have a code of ethics including unbiased reporting, providing context, ensuring accuracy, and vetting sources for credibility (Society of Professional Journalists, 2014).

Unbalanced Representation in Our Industry

Historically, journalists have not quoted nurses or other non-physician health care professionals in the news, even though these are news stories about topics that nurses and other health care professionals are very knowledgeable about. For example, The Woodhull study in 1997 found that nurses were referenced in health stories only 4% of the time (Sigma Theta Tau International, 1997), and that number has not improved. In 2017, 20 years later, Diana Mason, Laura Nixon, Barbara Glickstein, Sarah Han, Kristi Westphalm, and Laura Carter (2018) conducted a follow-up study. Still, nurses were not cited as expert sources; in a podcast interview, Diana Mason reported that things were worse—nurses were only named in 2% of health-related stories and none were related to health policy (Batchelor, 2020).

Why Is This?

There are multiple reasons; barriers such as newsroom editors who prefer physicians, communications leaders at our institutions who feed media requests to our physician colleagues first, and, of course, gender discrimination. Women, and women of color in particular, are not well represented in the media (Orenstein, 2020). Social media and your tenacity to be part of the conversation provides an opportunity to change this. We need to educate journalists and media outlet editors, and our organizational marketing and communication teams, on the value and expertise of all health care professionals.

Don't Be Afraid to Talk to Journalists

Journalists are people, too. They want the best information from the best sources to keep their audience's attention. This, again, is where owning your expertise and knowledge is the most important thing you should be thinking about. You've earned your place in the health care profession through your education, your practice, and your experience—now is the time for you to expand and share it with the world.

Prepare Your Elevator Speech

When talking to a journalist or a traditional media outlet, there are some basic rules of engagement.

Be Succinct

As with everything, you need to be able to make your point(s) quickly and with the least amount of unimportant information. You will lose your audience's attention if you drone on and on.

Don't Use Jargon

Your interview will likely be very short—and you won't have time to explain a lot of highly specialized terms. Try to minimize jargon, depending on your target audience. If your interview is going to be broadcast to the general public, use terms, metaphors, or stories to explain what you mean so that everyone can understand.

Think in Terms of Sound Bites

Prioritize and know your three main messages in terms of sounds bites. This will also help if you get nervous and forget all you wanted to say. Knowing your core messages in short sentences will help you remain focused and keep your interview on target.

We recommend a two-pronged approach for using social media to engage traditional media. The first is to use your available organizational resources like the marketing and/or media team and the second is to do it yourself.

Approach 1: Use Your Organization's Marketing and Media Teams

This may or may not surprise you, but your marketing and media relations teams are always looking for superstars to promote. In a large organization, it's hard to keep track of who does what. The media department ends up going back to the same people time and time again because they have met that expert source in person, have become familiar with them, and know they will do a good job representing the organization to fulfill the need of the reporter. But they also love to spread the wealth—the more experts an organization has to promote, the better the overall brand equity for the company in the public's eye. You have to initiate conversations with these marketing and media relations teams to let them know that you are available.

Lead With Your Brand

Make sure that the people who handle media and marketing know your name, your area of expertise, and any trending topics that might come up in the media. Set up a virtual meeting so you can see each other face-to-face and have a brief conversation. Prepare a summary of who you are and the credibility that you can lend to traditional media outlets looking for an expert source. Use your brand personality key words to make a stronger impression; be memorable. Once you have that first interaction with them, you're in. By nature of being their go-to person for a specific topic, they will contact you first for future media opportunities.

Nurture the Relationship

Marketing teams love building relationships. If you show that you are eager to help them do their job, they will work for you. They will create opportunities for you. Touch base with them every 6 months or so; tell them about the things you are doing. Don't be aggressive or demanding. Approach them in a way that furthers your relationship and brings them value, just like you do with your social media audience. Think about how you can both benefit from the situation and be in line with the needs of your organization. When you get a media placement, whether a quote or a feature, it's a win for everyone.

Be Ready for Them

Media requests can sometimes be made with only 1 hour's notice, so you need to be ready to drop what you're doing for a quick call with a reporter. If you're not available, the news source will move to the next person who is available. Your organization's media department should have your cell phone number, or email if you check it regularly, so you don't miss out on opportunities.

@MelissaBPhD

The media department at Melissa Batchelor's organization reached out when a reporter contacted them needing an expert to speak to "how to talk to your parents during COVID, and actually have them listen." This interview was published on CNBC Make It and led to an interview on NPR. The interview on NPR was heard by an individual who worked at Nasdaq. This individual reached out to her via LinkedIn and requested a presentation for Nasdaq's Employee Assistance Program on the same topic. This cascade of events and media shows the interconnection between how traditional and social media interact and demonstrates why having some presence on multiple platforms can be important if your email or phone number isn't public knowledge.

Google Yourself

If someone were looking to connect with you, what would they find if they Googled you? As you develop external professional relationships, bear in mind that reporters and media teams will check you out ahead of time. This is where all of the work you've done to develop your brand, hone your message(s), and your professional online/social media profile will solidify your expertise. All of these things help to establish your credibility, and now it's time to establish yourself as the go-to expert. Google yourself to see what comes up; this gives you an idea of what information would be shared with someone looking for you online.

For Better or For Worse

This is the state of today's digital world. You're better off knowing what pops up if you are Googled. There is a ton of public information online—from your property sales price, your marriage and divorce records, state salaries, names of relatives and previous addresses, even your age. With just a little bit of information on you (first name, occupation, place of work), you may be surprised at what comes up.

What to Do if You Don't Like What Comes Up

Sometimes you can reach out to the website to remove you or your associated account. You may want to keep different usernames for personal vs. professional accounts. If there is defamatory information online, you may have to resort to working with a company to help you remedy the situation. At the end of the day, it's better to know what comes up than not.

Social Can Also Be the Starting Point

We have found that when starting to promote their work, health care professionals who are active on social media first may have more success in traditional media outlets. This is because social media, especially Twitter, allows you to become comfortable expressing your own thought leadership. This allows your marketing team to get to know you and your work better—and make better connections for you with traditional media when a request for an expert comes in.

@APRNTerry

Terry Gallagher, a family nurse practitioner and assistant professor, started tweeting in 2018. Among other unique experiences, running a community clinic on the west side of Chicago gave her insight into the lives of underserved populations. Her tweets were views based on research and focused on how to make a difference in the lives of children and adults. Her strong brand personality resonated with her organization's marketing representatives who started noticing her work and how it was newsworthy. They reached out to her for promotional articles about her work to increase the organization's brand reputation and recruitment efforts. Dr. Gallagher transitioned to writing op-eds and had nine published in 1 year, which she then posted to her Twitter account. As a published author for *USA Today, U.S. News & World Report, The Hill, Chicago Tribune,* and featured on MSNBC, she became a trusted source for the media relations team. She always said yes. She personified her brand with reporters and interviewers. She is still called upon by her organization's media relations team for national and local television interviews for a wide range of topics because she established her expertise and advocacy through social media and op-ed writing.

@JBradyScott

Brady Scott, a respiratory therapist, started tweeting in 2017. As an associate professor, his enthusiasm for promoting the importance of respiratory care in the health system and as a career choice made his brand easy to recognize. He used skills learned in our Twitter workshop to create a network with colleagues and build his reputation. Naturally outspoken, Brady's passionate brand personality was contagious, and his organization's marketing team took notice. He started writing op-eds; the first was published in The Hill and earned 14,472 shares from the news site—the most direct site shares we have ever seen from an op-ed (Scott, 2019). In addition, exponential sharing happened when he, his professional respiratory care organization, and extended network also started posting the article link on Twitter, LinkedIn, and Facebook. When the COVID-19 pandemic started, the need for respiratory therapists was a trending topic in the news cycle. He was part of a unique team that started proning intubated patients to alleviate symptoms of the disease (Weiss et al., 2021). For this, and for his honest assessment of being a respiratory therapist during the pandemic, the media relations team selected him to be featured by CNN, Fox News, Associated Press, and countless other media outlets.

Both of these examples show how getting comfortable with publicly expressing yourself on social media translates to feeling comfortable transitioning to the traditional media arena. Finding and utilizing people and resources at your own organization is one way to guarantee support in connecting with journalists during this transition.

APPROACH 2: DO IT YOURSELF

Our second method for engaging traditional media through social media is to do it yourself. There are many strategies and online resources you can use to connect with journalists and news organizations and books to learn how to get media coverage (Daves, 2020).

Tag Journalists on Your Posts

Followerwonk is one of many tools you can use to find journalists and other influencers on Twitter. This tool aggregates key words from Twitter bios that are searchable. So, typing in "health reporter" in the search bar will give you a list of Twitter accounts who claim to be a health reporter in their bio.

Look up their Twitter profiles to see what they are all about. What types of stories do they write? Who do they usually use as sources, and how can you fit into that space or expand it? Once you do your research, don't be afraid to tag them if you're tweeting about a specific topic that you know they write about or if you have a compelling story that aligns with their realm and audience.

Use "Help A Reporter Out" (HARO) - @helpareporter

Follow this Twitter account made up of more than 75,000 journalists who have found 1.2 million sources for stories in top media outlets. A reporter posts what type of story they are writing and what type of source they are looking for. For instance: "#UrgHARO By 11pm ET: Seeking psychologists and sleep experts to comment on talking in your sleep. To reply, email query-b9jp@helpareporter.net" (Help A Reporter Out, 2020). When you see the #UrgHARO hashtag, it means the reporter is urgently seeking a source (Daves, 2020).

Writing an Op-Ed

Now we're getting deeper into the world of online influence. The term "op-ed" used to mean "opposite to the editorial page" in a newspaper, but today the term is used to mean an "opinion essay."

Writing an op-ed requires a completely different type of writing than you learned in your academic career. There is a structure and a cadence to opinion pieces, and if you start reading the op-ed section of any news outlet you can easily see the composition.

The OpEd Project - @theopedproject

We highly recommend using resources from TheOpEdProject.com for an introduction to writing these types of essays for digital publishing (The OpEd Project, n.d.). To master op-ed writing, we recommend taking a course from one of The OpEd Project's offerings. We all were trained by this organization, as were @APRNTerry and @JBradyScott in the earlier success stories. There are 1- and 2-day sessions that are open to the public for a fee. There are also year-long #PublicVoices fellowships for organizations willing to make a commitment for a diversified group of experts to tell their stories with the support of a high touch team of journalist mentors.

We believe, and know through tracking our organization's successes, that the work The OpEd Project is doing and the tools they offer are incredibly important for sharing your stories and insights with the world. To give you a taste of what is involved, here are five free tips from the website (The OpEd Project, n.d.).

5 Tips for Writing an Op-Ed

1. Don't bury the lede (or lead).
2. Think of an original idea about your area of expertise, or personal experience, and relate it to a news hook to catch attention.
3. Use data to support your argument.
4. Go to the bottom of news websites to find out where to send your op-ed draft.
5. Read published op-eds noting style and format.

Writing a Blog

If you don't want to wait for your topic to be published by someone else, you can always write a blog post. A blog is similar to an op-ed but doesn't need supporting data. Blogs are usually more personal in nature and can be published on LinkedIn, Facebook, or your own website or that of your organization.

References

Batchelor, M. (Host). (2020, April 13). Nurses representation in the media: An interview with Diana Mason (Episode No. 7) [Audiovisual Podcast]. In: *This is Getting Old: Moving Towards an Age-Friendly World*. https://bit.ly/3p7PXci

Daves, C. (2020). *The DIY guide to free publicity*. Monarch Crown Publishing.

Help a Reporter Out (HARO) [@helpareporter]. (2020, September 14). #URGHARO By 11pm ET: Seeking psychologists and sleep experts to comment on talking in your sleep. To reply, email query-b9jp@helpareporter.net [Tweet]. Twitter. https://bit.ly/2LCzHBJ

Mason, D., Nixon, L., Glickstein, B., Han, S., Westphaln, K., & Carter, L. (2018). The Woodhull study revisited: Nurses' representation in health news media 20 years later. *Journal Nursing Scholarship, 50*(6), 695-704. https://doi.org/10.1111/jnu.12429

Orenstein, K. (2020). *The OpEd Project Impact*. The Op Ed Project. https://bit.ly/3nLFh1U

Scott, J. B. (2019, October 25). *Respiratory therapists lead to better health outcomes*. The Hill. https://bit.ly/39EJ2ku

Sigma Theta Tau International. (1997). *The Woodhull study on nursing and the media: Health care's invisible partner. FINAL REPORT*. Center Nursing Press Sigma Theta Tau International. https://bit.ly/3oQLtra

Society of Professional Journalists. (2014, September 6). *SPJ code of ethics*. Society of Professional Journalists. https://bit.ly/3nLFh1U

The OpEd Project. (n.d.). *Op-ed writing: Tips and tricks*. The OpEd Project. https://bit.ly/2LAiEQL

Weiss, T. T., Cerda, F., Scott, J. B., Kaur, R., Sungurlu, S., Mirza, S. H., Alolaiwat, A. A., Kaur, R., Augustynovich, A. E., & Li, J. (2021). Prone positioning for patients intubated for severe acute respiratory distress syndrome (ARDS) secondary to COVID-19: A retrospective observational cohort study. *British Journal of Anaesthesia, 126*(1), 48-55. https://doi.org/https://doi.org/10.1016/j.bja.2020.09.042

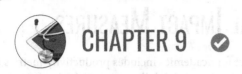

CHAPTER 9 ✔

Measuring Impact and Engagement

👍 Like   ↪ Share

♡   🗩   ⇄

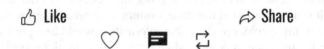

"Recognize that every interaction you have is an opportunity to make a positive impact on others."

Shep Hyken
@Hyken

Historically, measures of impact have been very narrow and primarily focused on measures important to those in the ivory tower. However, in today's world of technology and social media, academics and those engaged in health care scholarship are increasingly shifting their work to public-facing online platforms. Being able to translate your work and expertise into products that the public and policymakers can understand is becoming increasingly important. These new skills and methods of communication also mean alternative ways of capturing impact—measures beyond journal citation-based, article-level measures of impact, which may be primarily important for academics. Alternative metrics, broadly defined, are impact measures derived from various platforms and include tweets, retweets, downloads, website visits, number of views for blogs, podcasts, number of subscribers to YouTube Channels, comments on existing work, and inclusion in public policy discussions. You need to know about the different ways to measure impact and how to use both traditional and alternative metrics to measure the impact of your work.

Shattell, M., Batchelor, M., & Darmoc, R. *Social Media in Health Care:*
A Guide to Creating Your Professional Digital Presence (pp. 123-134).
© 2022 Taylor & Francis Group.

TRADITIONAL IMPACT MEASURES

Traditional measures of impact for academics includes productivity metrics such as number of publications and presentations, total dollar amount of grants, article citation rates, courses taught, and student evaluations of teaching effectiveness. And, of course, career advancement goals such as promotion and tenure.

For health care professionals in practice, pertinent metrics are usually those that are internal to the organization—patient outcomes, patient and staff satisfaction; number of patient days/visits per year; clinical ladders. External metrics include achieving and maintaining Magnet status and could expand to capturing community reach through your social media campaigns/posts and reviews on external websites. For example, if your organization has done a community needs assessment, creating microcontent or infographics to share that information would be a great way to extend public service and communication while building your local, regional, national, and international reputations as a leader in the field or specialty area.

For authors of scholarly publications, the impact of each publication or article is measured in number of citations, bookmarks, and mentions in social media, blogs, op-eds, and news articles. Citation-based metrics of impact include article level, journal level, and author level metrics.

Article-Level Metrics

Measuring impact at the article level is a bit more straightforward. You can easily use Scopus, Google Scholar, or other tools to see how many times an article was cited in the literature. Publishers can tell you how many page views and article downloads. And then tweets or mentions on other social media platforms that mention a particular article can also be tracked. Quotes in news articles and high-profile blogs are also good.

Journal-Level Metrics

Journal-level metrics include journal impact factor and rankings. Articles that are published in higher impact, more highly ranked journals have the potential to have greater impact.

Author-Level Metrics

Google Scholar Profile

If you have written and published anything (e.g., a scholarly paper, a commentary, a blog post, an op-ed) you should create a Profile in Google Scholar. Google Scholar captures your scholarly publications and gives you a list of them with the number of times each one has been cited. You can also click on the numbers to see who is citing your work. There will also be a graph by year and number of citations, and an overall total number of citations. This is essential for anyone who wants a traditional way to measure the impact of their work.

h-index

Academics who measure research and scholarship impact with traditional article-level metrics such as number of citations will also have a Scopus account (Scopus Preview, n.d.). In Scopus, you can see your h-index (x number of papers were cited at least x number of times; e.g., an h-index of 22 means that the person has 22 papers that have been cited at least 22 times). Where do these data come from? It depends on the source.

In Scopus, only academic/scholarly publications (articles) are counted toward the h-index. In Google Scholar, other digital content is included (e.g., non–peer-reviewed papers, op-eds, blogs) in addition to peer-reviewed articles and scientific/clinical presentations. Thus, depending on your audience, one might be more important than the other. It's because of this, that when asked (and people do), "what is your h-index?", we recommend giving both scores—your h-index from Scopus and your h-index from Google Scholar. It's just more clear.

ALTERNATIVE METRIC:
IMPACT BY SOCIAL MEDIA PLATFORM

A relatively easy way to show impact across all of the social media platforms is in the number of followers/friends/connections/subscribers. Impact on Facebook, Instagram, LinkedIn, Twitter, and YouTube can be measured by the number of followers, but more isn't necessarily better. It's better to have fewer, more engaged followers than hundreds of thousands of unengaged ones. Each platform has its own way to measure impact (Table 9-1).

Number of mentions is important anywhere in the digital environment. In Twitter, you want your content to get in front of more people, and this is called "impressions." In Twitter Analytics, you can see how many impressions each tweet has. You can also measure "engagement," which is the number of times a person interacts with your tweet (e.g., clicks on any of the links in your tweet). You can view the number of times your content is shared and reshared (retweets). You can see the comments on your content or replies to the replies. You can see how many people clicked into your content (e.g., if you post an article or a blog that you've written, and a person clicks on the article from the tweet, this is engagement).

TABLE 9-1. WAYS TO MEASURE IMPACT BY SOCIAL MEDIA PLATFORM

PLATFORM	MEASURES
FACEBOOK	Number of friends
	Number of mentions
	Engagement rate (the total number of engagements a post receives divided by the total number of impressions on that post)
TWITTER	Number of followers
	Number of mentions
	Number of tweets
	Number of clicks anywhere in the tweet (hashtags, embedded media, username, profile photo)
	Total engagements
	Total impressions
	Engagement rate (the total number of engagements a tweet receives divided by the total number of impressions on that tweet)
INSTAGRAM	Number of followers
	Number of posts
LINKEDIN	Number of connections in your network
YOUTUBE	Number of subscribers
	Number of views
OP-EDS/BLOGS	Per op-ed/blog post—number of views, shares, comments, likes
PODCASTS	Number of subscribers

Reciprocity Between Social and in Real Life (#IRL)

When you engage with social media, unexpected things can happen. Connections with potential collaborators can result in new and exciting projects that make a difference in (the) real lives of others (#IRL). New business relationships can result in new business opportunities. Networking in the social space can result in speaking engagements.

Opening Doors

Being present on social media may also improve your employment prospects. If the leader of a major organization is familiar with your professional online presence, and it is complementary to the mission and vision of their organization, they may just reach out to you. Being online creates a sense of familiarity with you and your work, whether or not you've met #IRL or not. Being perceived as reputable online can lead to engagement with leaders in the field who share, tweet, and comment on what you write—and could lead to being recruited.

ALTERNATIVE METRIC: ATTENTION

Attention metrics are measures of overall attention that an article attains. There are several but we will review the two most commonly known: Altmetrics and PlumX.

Altmetrics

Altmetrics was developed as a complement to the traditional measures of impact of scholarly work—the h-index and journal impact factors, which only track citations in scholarly journals. Altmetrics collects data from a wide variety of digital content (e.g., policy documents, newspapers, social media, blog posts and op-eds, mentions in traditional media, Wikipedia, citation software such as Mendeley and CiteULike) and result in an Altmetric attention score for each academic paper (Altmetric, 2020).

The algorithm calculates the score based on quantity and quality of attention. Many publishers (e.g., Wiley) now post Altmetric Attention Scores on the website for each article. Look for it—it's a colorful circle, with a numeric score in the middle of it. When you click on your Altmetric Attention Score, you will see the number of mentions, citations, and readers.

Altmetric Attention Score

Your Altmetric Attention Score can be found on the article page on the journal publisher's website under the Metrics section (Shattell et al., 2007). This metric allows you to see all sorts of information such as the countries where the readers are from (drawn from Mendeley and CiteULike), blog posts where the article is mentioned, citations in Wikipedia, news articles and outlets where the article was referenced, and even videos that discuss the article. The Altmetric Attention Score gives a much broader picture of how one's work is used and discussed in the public realm.

PlumX

Other publishers (e.g., Elsevier) use another metric, PlumX metrics, to calculate impact (Plum Analytics, 2020). Like Altmetrics, it uses more data, from a broad range of sources to calculate the impact of all types of scholarly research output. PlumX provides insight into how people are interacting with a variety of research products (e.g., articles, book chapters, conference proceedings).

PlumX tracks (1) citations, traditional citations such as in Scopus and other citations that indicate impact on society such as clinical or policy citations; (2) usage, determined by clicks, downloads, views to indicate if anyone is really using your research output; (3) captures, such as the number of bookmarks for the work as an indication that someone would want to revisit the research product at a later date; (4) mentions, measures activities related to any news article or blog post that mentions the work as an indicator of how much people are truly engaged with the work; and (5) social media, how many likes, tweets, and retweets to determine the amount of "buzz" and promotion a work is getting on social media platforms. Together this composite score gives a better overall view of impact—how people are truly using and interacting with a scholarly research product (Plum Analytics, 2020).

ALTERNATIVE METRIC: INDEX MEASURES

We will review the major index scores of impact across platforms and domains as of today. We know these metrics will change and newer ones will replace them. It's up to you to keep an eye out, to continue to explore newer ways to measure the impact of your work.

Symplur Healthcare Social Graph

Symplur is the only social media analytics company (that we are aware of) that is 100% focused on health care and health care influencers. In addition to finding health care–related hashtags and conference hashtags that are currently trending, you can use Symplur to find your Healthcare Social Graph score, which is an influencer score based on your Twitter activity with health care–related content (Symplur, n.d.).

It's Easy to Check

You first authorize Symplur Healthcare Social Media to access your Twitter account, and then a few moments later you'll get a webpage that shows your score (from 0 to 100), which is for the past 52 weeks' worth of data. You can also see your trends over time, in a graph, chart, and in numbers. You can also see how you compare to other health care influencers.

Followerwonk

We have mentioned Followerwonk because it's useful to search Twitter profiles when you are looking for influencers to follow. In addition to finding followers, Followerwonk also calculates an overall influencer score for each Twitter handle, which they call a "Social Authority" score (Bray, 2013). Social Authority is transparent, composed of the number of retweets a user has for the previous few hundred tweets, how recently those retweets occurred, and a retweet-based model developed to analyze user profile data (Bray, 2013). The overall score "is an amalgamation of follower count, tweets, the age of the account, and influence of followers ... a proprietary metric of Followerwonk" (Followerwonk, 2020).

These alternative and more broad-based measures of impact help researchers, health care professionals, and administrators know who is interacting with their work or brand, and how work is being promoted. Enhancing your digital presence and building a following in social media and other digital spaces gives you and your organization the opportunity to amplify your voice through public attention and engagement.

OTHER ALTERNATIVE METRICS

Media Monitoring

Do the number of times and the places where you and your work are mentioned equate to impact? Do you want to know when you are mentioned on the internet? There are several free and easy-to-use services. The two that we use are Google Alerts and Mention. There likely are others.

Google Alerts

Google Alerts are easy to use and will only take you approximately 2 minutes to set up. Shattell has alerts set up for variations configurations of her name (Mona Shattell, M. Shattell, M. M. Shattell). You can set this up to get daily emails with updates, or weekly if you prefer. It's really useful to know when and where your name shows up on the internet.

Mention

Another example is using the website Mention.com. You can track when your name is used on the web or on social media. Altmetric Attention Score tracks when an article is linked but might not mention your name. Thus, using Mention and your Altmetric Attention Score is important for more fully measure impact.

A GUIDE TO MEASURING SOCIAL MEDIA IMPACT BY THE 3C'S MODEL

Another way to think about your metrics is by the 3C's Model. These metrics will change over time as you continue on your social media journey. You can use them to measure in a variety of ways to demonstrate the impact of your work—for awards, promotions, annual evaluations, and future employment applications. You will need to put your metrics into context for your reader. These metrics are a powerful way to communicate how your online presence informs your professional activities and/or impact.

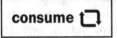

Following and Followers

Warning: Do not follow 6000 people and only have 6 followers. This is a clear indication that you just accepted random followers who are not necessarily interested in your content or your brand. When starting out on social media, keep these two numbers fairly balanced. Your goal is to follow others over time that you have a connection with and have them follow you back. You want to steadily grow the number that you follow and those who follow you over time. Having this as your primary metric is perfectly reasonable at this point.

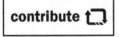

Following and Followers

This is still your primary metric, but now you begin to expand and monitor your impact by level of engagement with your followers.

Number of Likes and Retweets

Having an idea of the number of likes and retweets you are getting can help you gauge the level of interest in the posted topic by others. For some posts (and users), this may matter; for others, not so much. If you want to increase the number of likes and retweets you are getting, consider upping the level of engagement elicited by your posts by creating a poll, or asking an open-ended question rather than only making close-ended statements.

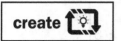

Following and Followers

Even at this level, this is still a primary metric to demonstrate your impact. If you're to go through the effort to Create original content, you should see continued growth over time per platform—depending on where your target audience is.

Overall Engagement Metrics

This includes everything—your total number of tweets and the number of likes, shares, retweets, and/or views.

How to Use the Metrics

To increase your level of engagement, use the engagement metrics to make decisions about future content. Making data-based decisions gleaned from your insights allows you to develop the content your target audience is most interested in.

Metrics Report Across Platforms

While not the primary driver for why you would want to be on social media, having an idea of your growth over time can be helpful. You should treat these numbers as a "personal best" rather than viewing them as a competition with others. We have provided an example of measuring metrics across time per platform for a campaign to raise awareness about ageism. Even with the goal of actively growing reach and impact, you can see the progress is slow, but steady. If that's your goal, the number one strategy to grow is consistently create new, value-added content that your audience is interested in (Table 9-2).

Measuring impact from traditional measures to social media index scores are both important. We recommend that you measure impact by the most common social media platforms you use and include the metrics as part of your professional social media plan(s). Use the data to propel you to the level you want to achieve. Your metrics should reflect your goals—whether that is to interact with a small number of professionals in your field or a large number of the public. Be consistent and persistent to raise any metric that fits your plan.

TABLE 9-2. SOCIAL MEDIA ACCOUNT PROFILE GROWTH

PLATFORM	JUNE	JULY	AUGUST	SEPTEMBER	OCTOBER	NOVEMBER
FACEBOOK	310 likes / 312 followers	338 likes / 343 followers	340 likes / 343 followers	341 likes / 345 followers	347 likes / 352 followers	351 likes / 361 followers
	223 average weekly post reach	315 average weekly post reach	248 average weekly post reach	237 average weekly post reach	73 average weekly post reach	66 average weekly post reach
	93 average weekly video views	160 average weekly video views	170 average weekly video views	109 average weekly video views	23 average weekly video views	35 average weekly video views
LINKEDIN	1300+ connections	1300+ connections	1500+ connections	1660+ connections	1660+ connections	1660+ connections
	169 viewed profile	162 viewed profile	157 viewed profile	173 viewed profile	156 viewed profile	125 viewed profile
	39 average post views	27 average post views	27 average post views	29 average post views	39 average post views	7 to 34 average post views
	19 search appearances	19 search appearances	19 search appearances	49 search appearances	57 search appearances	57 search appearances

(continued)

Table 9-2. Social Media Account Profile Growth (Continued)

PLATFORM	JUNE	JULY	AUGUST	SEPTEMBER	OCTOBER	NOVEMBER
TWITTER	1307 followers	1320 followers	1379 followers	1409 followers	1427 followers	1482 followers
	23 tweets (-25.8%)	11 tweets (-45%)	31 tweets (+29.2%)	19 tweets (-48.6%)	57 tweets (+185%)	31 tweets (-48.3%)
	21.3K impressions (+53.6%)	5.89K impressions (-67.8%)	15.3K impressions (+47%)	12.4K impressions (-19.1%)	23.2K impressions (+97%)	26K impressions (-0.8%)
	139 profile visits (+17.6%)	76 profile visits (-49.7%)	377 profile visits (+135.6%)	274 profile visits (-34.3%)	209 profile visits (-19.3%)	444 profile visits (+85.8%)
	37 mentions (+236.4%)	10 mentions (-49.7%)	13 mentions (-35%)	19 mentions (+5.6%)	39 mentions (+85.7%)	19 mentions (-50%)
INSTAGRAM	257 followers / 230 posts	279 followers / 254 posts	286 followers / 286 posts	288 followers / 311 posts	298 followers / 311 posts	308 followers / 362 posts
	9 average weekly posts	9 average weekly posts	6 average weekly posts	6 average weekly posts	5 average weekly posts	5 average weekly posts
	1267 average impressions	1111 average impressions	1111 average impressions	920 average impressions	668 average impressions	629 average impressions

REFERENCES

Altmetric. (2020, September 17). *How is the Altmetric attention score calculated?* Altmetric. https://bit.ly/3azk1to

Arora, A., Bansal, S., Kandpal, C., Aswani, R., & Dwivedi, Y. (2019, July 1). Measuring social media influencer index- insights from facebook, Twitter and Instagram. *Journal of Retailing and Consumer Services, 49*, 86-101. https://doi.org/https://doi.org/10.1016/j.jretconser.2019.03.012

Bray, P. (2013, February 13). *Social authority: Our measure of Twitter influence.* Moz. https://bit.ly/37vtyiZ

Followerwonk (2020, September 22). *Frequently asked questions.* Followerwonk. https://bit.ly/383rtO7

Plum Analytics. (2020). *About PlumX metrics.* Plum Analytics. https://bit.ly/34s9qfV

Scopus Preview. (n.d.). *Welcome to Scopus preview.* Elsevier. https://bit.ly/34wmuRs

Shattell, M. M., Starr, S. S., & Thomas, S. P. (2007). "Take my hand, help me out": Mental health service recipients' experience of the therapeutic relationship. *International Journal of Mental Health Nursing, 16*(4), 274-284. https://doi.org/10.1111/j.1447-0349.2007.00477.x

Symplur. (n.d.). *Look up your healthcare social graph score.* Symplur. https://bit.ly/2Wxr3Xk

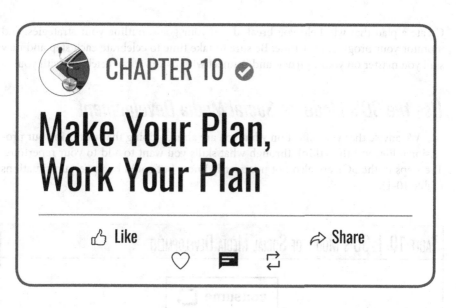

CHAPTER 10 ✓

Make Your Plan, Work Your Plan

👍 Like   ↪ Share

♡   💬   ⇄

> "If you're prepared and you know what it takes, it's not a risk. You just have to figure out how to get there. There is always a way to get there."
>
> *Mark Cuban*
> *@mcuban*

If you were going to take a hike, you would be sure to have a map, compass, or some other type of navigation tool with you to ensure that you didn't get lost in the woods. Having a clear sense of direction means you won't miss the forest for the trees. The same is true for planning your professional impact using social media. Look at the work products you are already creating (e.g., traditional publications, presentations, posters) and focus on re-envisioning that work into a format that can be shared with a wider audience. Be sure to incorporate your professional brand as you Consume, Contribute, and Create content to share with the digital world.

BABY STEPS

Moving forward using social media takes time and attention, but it shouldn't overwhelm your life. Start with a vision and plan for how you would like to develop your skills over time. Think of this as planning for a marathon—not a sprint.

Shattell, M., Batchelor, M., & Darmoc, R. *Social Media in Health Care: A Guide to Creating Your Professional Digital Presence* (pp. 135-154).

Create a plan that will help you break down your goals, outline your strategies, and monitor your progress over time. Be sure to take time to celebrate each step and new skill you master on your journey, and connect with us so we can celebrate with you!

Use the 3C's Model of Social Media Development

We advise that you reflect on what you are already doing that works in your professional life, and then think through what skills you want to add to your repertoire. The steps in the 3C's are also not necessarily linear but could be in certain situations (Table 10-1).

TABLE 10-1. 3C's MODEL OF SOCIAL MEDIA DEVELOPMENT

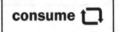

- Learn new social media platform, educate family and friends (like, share, retweet without comment)

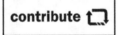

- Interpreting health information and translating it for the public (retweet with comment, blogging, op-eds, sharing conference events [within social media rules])

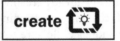

- Advocacy, thought leadership (podcast, TV/radio, meeting with policymakers, original video content)

PLANNING PHASES

The following content will take you through the process of developing three types of plans that could be worked on in a linear manner or mixed and matched, depending on your goals and message.

As you review these phases and types of planning, remember that you can make them as simple or as complex as you would like. We will present them at various levels, so you can see the differences.

Phase 1: Decision-Making and Prioritization

We recommend starting this process with making some decisions and prioritizing what skills you need to develop first. Once you are comfortable as a Consumer and Contributor, if it fits your goal(s), move into creating your own content and develop a plan to disseminate your content to have the greatest possible impact (Table 10-2; Box 10-1).

Phase 2: Professional Development Plan

A professional development plan can help you prioritize development of your social media skills over time and lay out your vision for flipping your traditional work products into innovative products for dissemination (Table 10-3; Figure 10-1).

Phase 3: Social Media Implementation Plan

This can be used to guide dissemination across platforms. This plan can be simple or complex, depending on what you want to share and with whom (Table 10-4; Figure 10-2).

Phase 4: Content Creation Plan

At this level, you've hit the big leagues! Now you begin to strategize about what content you want to Create and when (Table 10-5).

ROADMAP FOR PHASE 1:
DECISION-MAKING AND PRIORITIZATION

The first step in your own development starts with answering a few questions about your own professional priorities and how you can repurpose what you are already doing into a new product for social media. Once you have these answers, you can move forward. Creating a sequenced plan based on time, energy, interest, and available resources is critical for helping to move you through the social media maze. Adding individual steps can help you recognize progress over time—which may be what you need to motivate yourself to take it to the next level.

What Do You Want to Get Out of Social Media?

Answering this question first will help keep you focused and on track. When you begin your professional social media journey with the end in mind, it will help you create an efficient and effective plan to make sure you arrive at your intended destination. The answer to this question also drives how you prioritize skill development and what resources it will take to achieve your goal.

What Is Your Specific Goal?

While there are many reasons to use social media, being very clear about your own specific goal is a critical first step. You may already be on social media to maintain personal connections with family and friends, but you will need to make conscious decisions about which social media you would like to use professionally. You will also need to decide which platforms you would like to use personally and which ones (if any) blend your personal and professional lives.

What Is Your Main Message?

What is your area of expertise and what content do you want to share? As you developed your brand, you should have zeroed in on the things you are most known for. Your area of expertise is how you will derive what your core message will be when you are creating content, but you will likely also be led to follow people within your business to Consume and Contribute to the thoughts and ideas they are posting.

Who Is Your Target Audience?

Know your audience, but also let them get to know you. While social media is online, you want your audience to develop an emotional attachment to you, your brand, your business, and/or your messages. Encouraging your audience to engage in the online conversation and make it their own is one way to help build this emotional attachment.

Media/Social Media Outlet of Choice?

Once you have decided who your target audience is, this information will guide which social media platform you may want to use. For example, we recommend that you begin your journey using free platforms and apps to amplify your voice. Based on your goals, message, and target audience, you may eventually move into needing your own website to serve as a living curriculum vitae—a one-stop shop for compiling your blog, videos, podcasts, publications, presentations, recent news or events, honors or awards, and links for how your audience can connect with you (e.g., subscribe to your email listserv, subscribe to your YouTube Channel, follow you on social).

What Skills Do You Need to Execute Your Plan?

Be a lifelong learner. Each of us started somewhere. Over the years, we have developed expertise by exploring something new and testing it to see if it fits our own goals. We experienced successes and failures but over time we have each found our niche in the social media landscape. When a new social media outlet is released, we have each taken a little time to explore it and see how others are using it before we make a commitment. Being flexible and open to change is a good strategy because you will have to go where your target audience goes if one platform disappears.

What Resources Are Needed?

You can fully engage with social media for free and still be a major leader/influencer in your field. Expenses don't typically exceed more than your time, effort, and energy until you have a goal to create content that is widely disseminated across multiple social media platforms and potentially into podcast platforms like iTunes, Spotify, Stitcher, and Amazon Music. Uploading the content to most of these platforms is free, it will just take time (and time is money!). As you advance, you will be best served to identify a team that can help you be successful. Trying to do all of this on your own is often too much for one person unless it's your full-time job.

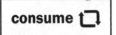

Consuming social media takes the least amount of time, effort, and energy. We have busy personal and professional lives, so check in when it's convenient for you to get news and information from those you follow. When you think about social media as an integrated part of your life, it makes it easier to engage with (in some cases) than thinking about it as "I need to spend 1 hour every day on social media." Integrating social media into your life, to us, means using the "down time" of life more efficiently.

Using Down Time

Use the time spent standing in line or commuting to catch up on recent activities. We find this to be an easier way to stay connected without it feeling like an overwhelming task. Consuming social media is also the least expensive level and requires the least amount of support.

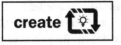

Contributing to social media may take slightly more time than consuming, but it is the next level when you are moving toward thought leadership. For these reasons, learning to Contribute is also an inexpensive level and doesn't typically require a lot of support. This is a strategy we use as an integral part of practicing the 80-20 rule.

80-20 Rule

Remember approximately 80% of your activity on social is sharing posts from other people. This can be as simple as clicking the retweet button on Twitter or the share button from an online article. You can easily find time in your day to do this once or twice, so don't overthink it and let it overwhelm you.

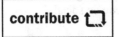

When you begin to Create your own content, this is where expenses can come in. This step is largely driven by how much time, effort, and energy you have to devote to a social media project or strategy and what your ultimate goal is with your work. You may need to learn new skills, but you can gain these skills through friends, family, or free demonstration videos on YouTube. You can also use the Apple Educator online and face-to-face courses to learn how to use KeyNote, GarageBand, and/or iMovie (Apple Inc., 2020).

Table 10-2. Decision-Making and Prioritization

WHAT DO YOU WANT TO GET OUT OF SOCIAL MEDIA?	RESOURCES
What is your specific goal?	Time, effort, and energy to develop your professional plan for using social media at each developmental level • Consume • Contribute • Create
What is your main message?	Time, effort, and energy to develop your plans for content creation and social media implementation
Who is your target audience?	Following others and organizations and building your following in the platforms most relevant to your target audience
Media/social media outlet choice?	Free platforms: Consume, Contribute, and Create • YouTube • Twitter • Facebook • Instagram • LinkedIn Funding: Create • Equipment: Smartphone, tablet or laptop to record video and/or take photos • Creating graphics: Canva, Unsplash (both free) • Website (or use home institution resources): Domain name for website (GoDaddy and others); WordPress, Squarespace, Wix, Bootstrap, and others (some are free or you pay to upgrade); Virtual Assistant/Website Builder/Website Maintenance; MailChimp (or some other email listserv service) • Blog: LinkedIn, WordPress • Podcast (audio and video): Podcast platform (Lisbyn); equipment (lighting, microphone, camera or smartphone, laptop, backdrop)

(continued)

Table 10-2. Decision-Making and Prioritization (continued)

WHAT DO YOU WANT TO GET OUT OF SOCIAL MEDIA?	RESOURCES

What skills do you need to execute your plan?	Skill development (with a few examples)
	• Consume
	   o Identify most effective platform for professional use
	   o Create your profile
	   o Optimize your bio
	   o Follow relevant people and organizations
	• Contribute
	   o Build your following
	   o Learn to retweet
	   o Learn to retweet with comment
	   o Learn to use #hashtags and @handles effectively
	• Create
	   o Learn to create original posts with graphic/video
	   o Use #hashtags and @handles effectively
	   o Create original content in the form of graphics, infographics, video, or live streaming
	   o Organize Twitter chats
	Funding: Support
	• Production
	   o Do-it-yourself
	   o Outsource to a production company
	Funding: Dissemination
	• Hootsuite
	   o Do-it-yourself
	   o Outsource to a virtual assistant

Box 10-1. Answer the Following Questions to Help You Stay Focused	
GOAL	
MAIN MESSAGE	
TARGET AUDIENCE	
MEDIA OR SOCIAL MEDIA OUTLET	
PROFESSIONAL CONTENT TO SHARE	
WHAT SKILLS DO YOU NEED TO EXECUTE?	
WHAT RESOURCES ARE NEEDED?	

Roadmap for Phase 2: Crafting Your Professional Development Plan

When you are first getting started in social media, it's helpful to Create a professional development plan. This helps you to organize what platform you will begin to learn more about first, develop the skills for using that platform proficiently, and then begin to Create your own content to share your expertise. Pick and choose what will give you the most "bang for your buck" rather than thinking of this as a linear process—because we each have 24 hours in a day, and you can't do everything all at once, by yourself.

Building Your Professional Social Network

For those of you who are just getting started, we recommend prioritizing building your professional social network first. We also recognize that this may be the highest and only priority for many people—it is a laudable goal and where each of us started! You can make a huge impact through your connections and adding your own thoughts to any online dialogue. Spend some time in this phase to build your basic social media skills before moving on to develop an advanced professional development plan.

Flipping Products

We have found it helpful to start with what you know and examine what you are already doing before you get started. Most professionals are doing some level of traditional dissemination, so begin to think about products, such as a blog (examples from Table 10-3) you have already created and decide what innovative dissemination products you may be able to Create and what dissemination platforms would work best to get your message out (see Figure 10-1).

SMART Goals

We recommend setting SMART goals (Box 10-2) and keeping them in a place where you can see them (Copeland, n.d.). SMART goals are:

- Specific goal (what innovative product do you want to create from prior work)
- Metrics (how impact will be measured)
- Achievable (how much time/what resources are needed to execute this goal)
- Relevant audience (who do you want to receive your message + platform)
- Timeline (what time frame do you want to achieve this goal within? [e.g., 1 to 3 months])

TABLE 10-3. PROFESSIONAL DEVELOPMENT PLAN

BUILD YOUR PROFESSIONAL SOCIAL NETWORK

PLATFORM	WHAT DO YOU DO ALREADY?	WHAT WOULD YOU LIKE TO DO IN THE NEXT MONTH?	WHAT WOULD YOU LIKE TO DO IN THE NEXT 6 MONTHS?
Facebook	Personal page to connect with family	Create a professional Facebook Page for my research	Join Facebook Groups that relate to my research and interact with members (e.g., caregiver groups)
Instagram	Personal account to share photos		
Twitter		Consume and Contribute Goals: Follow 10 people/organizations per week; five retweets per week	Create by adding my own thought leadership to other tweets and articles Goal: One original tweet per week
LinkedIn		Edit my bio, photo, experience, & awards to ensure my profile is aligned with my brand and expertise	"Connect" with nursing/academic professionals Goal: 100 connections in 6 months
TRADITIONAL PRODUCTS	*WHAT DO YOU DO ALREADY?*	*WHAT WOULD YOU LIKE TO DO IN THE NEXT MONTH?*	*WHAT WOULD YOU LIKE TO DO IN THE NEXT 6 MONTHS?*
Publications		Promote my most recent publication on Twitter with link to the article and tweeting a short summary	Post additional content/ knowledge about my publication's implications
Presentations	Poster presentation	Create a 1-minute video abstract for my poster presentation	Share my 1-minute video on a social media platform

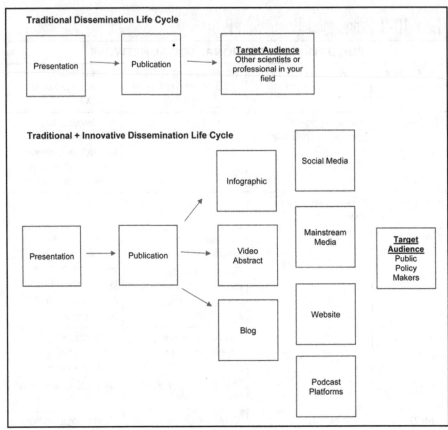

Figure 10-1. Traditional vs. innovative products for dissemination.

Box 10-2. SMART Goal	
SPECIFIC GOAL	
METRIC (IMPACT)	
ACHIEVABLE	
RELEVANT AUDIENCE	
TIMELINE	

ROADMAP FOR PHASE 3:
PLANNING A SOCIAL MEDIA CAMPAIGN

Once you have your content created and skills to manage a few social media platforms, the next step is creating your own social media campaign (i.e., social media marketing strategy).

In the example that we share, the social media campaign was designed for a long -form podcast video disseminated on social media (see Table 10-4). It is a high-level plan to disseminate original content, but we have included it so that you can see the various steps and tailor it to fit your goals. You can simplify the plan by focusing on one platform, creating one post, and using only one image/graphic per week. You can step it up later by adding a second platform, microcontent video(s), blogs, and/or additional microcontent videos and graphics.

Tailor to the Platform

Post

These are either long- or short-form depending on the platform. You can say more on Facebook, LinkedIn, and Instagram, but need to stay within the 280-character limit for Twitter. It is best practice to slightly change your posts from platform to platform, and posting on multiple platforms will increase engagement with your audience.

Names, Handles, and Hashtags

When you are creating a social media campaign, you will need to tailor not only your word/character limit, but also the tags, hashtags, and handles to each platform depending on the topic and your target audience.

TIME SAVER TIP

Use a social media posting and scheduling tool like Hootsuite or Tweet Deck to schedule your posts in advance. You select the date/time for your post and the tool will post for you. This allows you to create several posts in one time block, rather than trying to post something in real-time every few days. Your content will continue to come out according to your schedule, but you're not spending every day organizing and posting to multiple platforms.

Metrics

You will also want to use metrics to make data-based decisions for these campaigns based on your goal and objectives.

TABLE 10-4. SOCIAL MEDIA IMPLEMENTATION PLAN

FACEBOOK/LINKEDIN

In this week's This Is Getting Old Show, I talked about 10 warning signs that you should look out for if you're concerned about someone's memory. The first warning sign is that the memory problem is significant enough that it impacts the person's ability to take care of themselves every day.

Tune into the full episode to learn the other nine warning signs of Alzheimer's disease (Figure 10-2). It's likely not what you think. https://melissabphd.com/podcastblog/

LINKEDIN AND FACEBOOK HASHTAGS AND HANDLES

@Alzheimer'sAssociation® @Alzheimer'sSociety
@Alzheimer'sAssociationCorporatePartnerships @Alzheimer'sCareManagement
@Alzheimer'sAssociationWNYChapterEvents
@'ADS'DementiaAwarenessTrainingintheCommunity @Alzheimer'sWA
@AmericanNursesAssociation #nurseschangelives #nursesonlinkedin

INSTAGRAM

In this week's This Is Getting Old Show, I talked about 10 warning signs that you should look out for if you're concerned about someone's memory. The first warning sign is that the memory problem is significant enough that it interrupts the person's ability to take care of themselves every day.

Tune into the full episode to learn the other nine warning signs of Alzheimer's disease. It's likely not what you think. Click the link in the bio. @alzassociation @alzheimerssoc @alzheimerspodcast

INSTAGRAM HASHTAGS:

#alzheimersawareness #alzheimers #alzheimerssucks #alzheimersassociation #alzheimerscare #alzheimersscare #alzheimersawarenessmonth #alzheimersdisease #alzheimerssociety #alzheimerscaregiver #alzheimerssupport #alzheimerswarningsigns

TWITTER

Are you concerned that your loved one has early signs of #Alzheimers? Tune into this week's episode of This Is Getting Old podcast—"Ten Signs of Alzheimer's Disease." https://melissabphd.com/podcastblog/ #olderadults #Dementia #forget #memoryproblems

TWITTER HASHTAGS AND HANDLES

@EndALZ #alzheimersawareness #alzheimers #alzheimerssucks #alzheimersassociation #alzheimerscare #alzheimersscare #alzheimersawarenessmonth #alzheimersdisease #alzheimerssociety #alzheimerscaregiver #alzheimerssupport #alzheimerswarningsigns

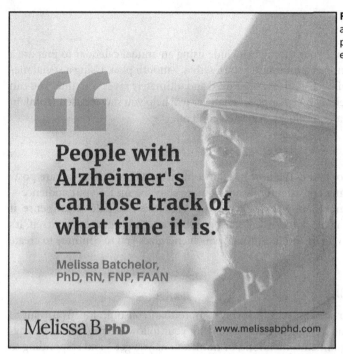

Figure 10-2. Graphic to accompany social media post related to a full episode.

ROADMAP FOR PHASE 4: PLANNING CONTENT CREATION

Creation is the highest level of social media engagement and isn't for the faint of heart. Moving into content creation can be nerve wracking—but also very exciting! In general, start with a time frame that is achievable so you aren't overwhelmed (see Table 10-5).

Quality Over Quantity

Your focus here should be on quality, not quantity. Posting quality content once every month (or once every quarter) is better than trying to produce something every week that falls flat. Start with a reasonable goal—our philosophy is that it's always easier to increase content production over time than become frustrated that you aren't meeting your goals.

Get Organized

Options to organize your thoughts include using an annual calendar to prepare a theme for your content—at a minimum, start with a 3-month plan. Using a social media content planner will help you stay organized and ultimately saves you time. You can use a paper-based or electronic planner—whatever will help you stay focused. Think in terms of monthly themes or blocks of related content.

Be Consistent

Another benefit of taking the time to plan content is to ensure that you are posting consistently. Posting consistently means you are showing up for your audience—whether once every month, bi-weekly, or weekly. While this rationale makes sense, it can also be a stumbling block to getting started. Set an attainable goal for yourself. It's better to make smaller goals and meet them, which energizes you to continue to create content.

Build Community

To be a leader in social media, it involves more than consumption. You want to build a community and develop a relationship with your followers. You do this by paying attention to the comments, mentions, or notifications you get—and responding to them.

Content Ideas

Trend Overview

You are the expert in your field, or at least a very informed health care professional on a given topic. What are the trends in your area that you think would be of interest to the public and/or consumers of health care information? Identifying trends in mainstream media, social media, and your professional networks (e.g., email, conference themes) are one good way to determine content for the month. If you want to plan in advance, using alternative content planning categories can be helpful. Otherwise, keeping a pulse on health information trends can determine what content you want to share for a given time frame.

Create Series

One way to develop content is around core themes such as telemedicine, population health, biometric devices, burnout, research, education, clinical practice, health policy, or trending leadership skills. Within each of these themes or special series, you can create original content and/or hosted interviews with experts in the field.

How-To Guides—Things to Know

How-To Guides give instructions for how to do something. In the health care arena, you may also want to conceptualize this as Things to Know. This is where you can really let your expertise shine vs. in an interview or profile, where you're highlighting the expertise of others. To get started, you could think about the things people typically ask you. Any patterns to these questions and your answers may provide insight on a given topic.

Interview/Profile

You don't always have to do the heavy lifting by going solo in content creation. Doing interviews and posting profiles of leaders in your field is also a great way to promote the work of others (remember the 80-20 rule).

Predictions

One example of predictions can be around the New Year (e.g., Things Hospitals Should Be Planning for in the Next 10 Years). If the majority of news for upcoming trends is focused on technology and hospitality trends for the acute care setting, maybe your angle is to create content related to how hospitals should be paying attention to becoming an age-friendly health system. This gives you an opportunity to make a unique contribution.

News

Consuming news is easy enough for anyone to do, but sharing news that comes across your desk is another great way to Contribute to the conversation via social media. This could come in the form of new reports, new evidence-based clinical practice guidelines, and/or tagging relevant mainstream media news with a comment that puts the news into perspective. You can also create your own news by alerting your media office to a recent publication.

Table 10-5. Content Creation Plan				
TIMELINE	**THEME/TOPIC**	**INNOVATIVE PRODUCT**	**PRODUCT PLATFORM**	**TITLE**
MONTH				
Week 1	Holiday	Blog + Infographic	Facebook + LinkedIn	Older Americans Month
Week 2	Raising awareness	Video	YouTube	Ten Signs of Alzheimer's Disease
Week 3	Interview/profile	Video + blog	YouTube + website	AHRQ Project Echo National Nursing Home COVID-19 Action Network— Interview with Dr. Alice Bonner
Week 4	Future prediction	Blog	Website	Top Five Future Trends in Health Care
MONTH				
Week 1	Age-friendly initiatives	Video + blog	YouTube + website	Age-Friendly Ecosystem
Week 2		Graphic	Twitter	Age-Friendly Cities and States
Week 3		Interview	Facebook Live	Age-Friendly Health Systems
Week 4		News	Instagram, LinkedIn, Facebook, and Twitter	Age-Friendly Public Health

ALTERNATIVE CONTENT PLANNING

Flipping Traditional Products

Any time you do a traditional poster or podium presentation, be thinking about what innovative dissemination product you could flip it into and how to best share with a broader audience.

Use Calendars

Be creative and make the connections for your audience. We each have a unique perspective, and this is one way to let that shine through.

Traditional Holidays

Most of us are aware of the traditional holiday calendar. If any of these relate to your work, take the opportunity to create and highlight related content.

Thanksgiving

If your work is focused on improving nutritional outcomes for older adults, you could write a blog for Thanksgiving, given that this holiday is strongly focused around the Thanksgiving meal and family traditions. If your work is focused on cardiovascular health, creating content for Valentine's Day is a natural fit—but you could also reframe content for the Thanksgiving holiday given the number of Turkey Trots many communities host on Thanksgiving morning.

Wacky Calendar

You can also check out Wacky Holiday Calendars to generate ideas for content (timeanddate.com, n.d.).

Pistachio Day

For February 26, you could create a post around how nuts are part of a heart-healthy diet—or a post raising awareness of nut allergies.

Relaxation Day

Depending on your area of expertise, you could create a graphic and post around mindfulness, burnout, how to use a biometric device to practice breathing, or encourage people to take up yoga.

CONCLUSION

Having a clear vision of what skills you need to develop and a "map" of your most important messages will help you navigate your own social media journey. These are just some ideas and examples to get your started in moving through the 3C's Model of Social Media Development. We hope you will also take the time to celebrate and share your small (and big) wins along the way.

REFERENCES

Apple Inc. (2020). *Apple Teacher.* https://apple.co/37CIHyW

Batchelor, M. (Host). (2020, June 24). Ten signs of alzheimer's disease (Episode 17) [Audiovisual podcast]. In: *This is Getting Old: Moving Towards an Age-Friendly World.* https://bit.ly/2WAQTcE

Batchelor, M. (Host). (2021, January 11). AHRQ ECHO National Nursing Home COVID-19 Action Network (Episode 44) In: *This is Getting Old: Moving Towards an Age-Friendly World.* https://bit.ly/2MXdTkC

Copeland, B. (n.d.). *SMART goals: How to make your goals achievable.* MindTools. https://www.mindtools.com/pages/article/smart-goals.htm

timeanddate.com. (n.d.). *Fun holidays - Funny, random & weird holidays.* timeanddate.com. https://bit.ly/3oFczkq

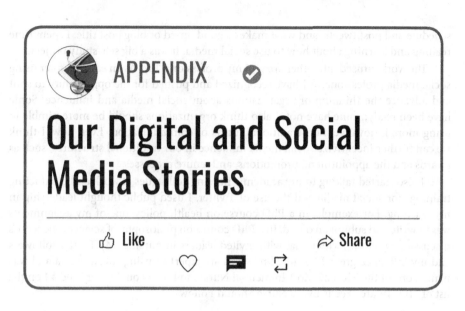

APPENDIX ✓

Our Digital and Social Media Stories

👍 Like   ↪ Share

♡   💬   ⇄

MONA

I started out slowly. As many people do. I was introduced to Twitter when I was in the Op-Ed Project Public Voices Fellowship program in 2012 as a professor at DePaul University. I had heard of Twitter but hadn't had an account and didn't really know much about it or what it could do. I had used Facebook for a long time but mostly for personal reasons—getting and staying connected with family and friends. I had not used social media in my professional life. But, during that session on public thought leadership in social media, my fellow participants and I were told about Twitter. Those of us who did not have accounts were encouraged to create one. That day, I created a Twitter account and began my foray into using social media to engage my professional life.

I started by following my fellow interdisciplinary Op-Ed Project participants, my academic nursing colleagues and friends, the organizations that I belonged to, and the main news outlets that I liked. I posted very little in those days. I mostly consumed information. I followed and read and retweeted posts that I thought were interesting. I was writing a lot during those years. I had a regular blog on HuffPost and wrote several op-eds and blogs with colleagues. I was learning about how and when to use social media to share the work. Simple Google searches revealed tips like when was the best time to post a tweet, what platform to use to

Shattell, M., Batchelor, M., & Darmoc, R. *Social Media in Health Care: A Guide to Creating Your Professional Digital Presence* (pp. 155-158).

schedule and post tweets, and what makes a good op-ed or blog post title. I spent time reading and learning about how to use social media. It was a big self-study project.

The work infused into other areas of my professional life. As an early adopter using social media professionally, I have recognized and pushed for the opportunity to shift and advance the thinking of organizations about social media and influence. Some have been ready; some have not. I also think organizations should be more nimble in using more innovative, non-traditional forms of communication. Even now, I think we can further incentivize social media influence in our traditional structures, such as awards and the appointment, promotions, and tenure processes.

I also started talking to my academic nursing colleagues at work and conducting trainings for social media and the use of Twitter. I used public thought leadership in my teaching. For example, in a PhD course on health policy, one of my assignments was to write and submit an op-ed. In a PhD course on philosophy of science, one week's discussion was as a Twitter chat with invited leaders in nursing. My Twitter followers and my influence grew. I became known as an expert in using social media and was named one of the "Top 25 Most Influential Nurses to Follow on Twitter" and #4 on the list of "100 Twitter Feeds Every Nurse Should Follow."

Melissa

The overarching goal of my health care career has always been to improve the quality of care delivered to older adults, especially those living with Alzheimer's disease in nursing homes. There was so much that people didn't know, and I wanted to help.

I started using social media with a personal Facebook account around 2005, mostly to keep in touch with family and friends. In 2009, I attended a leadership conference communications training and was encouraged to create a Twitter account. While I was comfortable with Facebook, Twitter was a mystery. Everything seemed to be written in hieroglyphics with these new #hashtags and @handles. I created my account, but it sat there for several years unattended.

In 2005, I also moved into nursing education to reach nurses at the beginning of their careers to share with them that a career in geriatrics was not only viable—it was exciting! Eager to learn ways to engage students with geriatric nursing content and as an avid podcast listener, I learned to record my classroom lectures as podcasts. In 2009, I had the opportunity to pitch the idea of turning the nine lectures that were part of the Geriatric Nursing Education Consortium into podcasts (Aselage, 2010). Over the next 5 years, the podcasts were accessed more than 60,000 times in more than 40 countries. This got my attention about the power of digital technology and metrics—given that 60,000 people were unlikely to read my traditional peer-reviewed publications.

I was attending a national conference years later and noticed people were using Twitter on a larger scale. This prompted me to dust off my old Twitter account and at least try to use Twitter. I asked someone to explain the hashtags and handles to me—and once I understood that the concepts for tweeting were similar to Facebook—to use handles as nouns to "tag" people and use hashtags as "adjectives"—I could construct a tweet! I slowly began to follow organizations and leaders in my field, but still primarily used Twitter when I attended conferences. At this point, I primarily consumed social media and would Contribute by retweeting with a comment.

In the spring of 2017, I had the opportunity to record seven public access television shows that were initially aired live, but also recorded and posted on YouTube. I thought it was unlikely for my social media audience to watch a 1-hour show, but I thought they might watch four 13-minute segments. I also show breaking up the show content as an opportunity to learn to develop a blog post for each shorter segment. Using the shorter segments of the show allowed me to release content on a weekly basis. I created a professional Facebook Page; ramped up my LinkedIn, Twitter, and Instagram accounts; and learned how to use Hootsuite. Hootsuite allowed me to schedule the content releases in one block of time after recording the show, but the content rolled out weekly across my platforms without any more time, energy, or effort on my part. This still took more time than I wanted it to, and I was constrained by having to be at the television studio in the evening once a month. I also wasn't quite sure I was doing the social media campaign correctly. The television shows ended as I began my Health and Aging Policy Fellowship in the fall of 2017, but I continued to use social media in a professional capacity, and the seed had been planted for what I might want to do next.

In 2019, I connected with a podcast production company at a conference and began a podcast series in March of 2020. I also knew I needed to hire a Virtual Assistant if I wanted to maximize my impact. With this new setup, I have been able to record the podcast content from home using Zoom, which also allows me to interview others and create content at any point in my day/week that works for me. Once recorded, I send the video to the production company who develops the blog, graphics, microcontent, and the social media implementation plan for my four platforms. After the production company is finished with each of these products, they are passed along to my Virtual Assistant who schedules them to go out for me and posts them into four podcast platforms. This means content is coming out weekly, and microcontent comes out three times a week. I'm still learning, as we all are, but continue to see the impact of developing quality niche content on a consistent basis to help older adults and their families.

REBECCA

I am an introvert. One might think this is a conundrum for getting involved in social media, but I'd like to share why it is not a disqualifier and how social media has enhanced my life.

Social media became more popular from 2000 to 2010. I was in my mid-20's and Facebook was taking over the world. As an introvert, the last thing I wanted to do was share pictures, plans, or other personal information with a large group of people. It gave me hives just thinking about it. But all my friends were doing it so I joined Facebook just to see what I was missing. I was missing a lot. Eventually I started participating instead of watching; it was fun to banter back and forth with my real friends on this platform and share fun aspects of my life—like a video of an epic dance-off at a wedding we all attended. The one thing I appreciated about Facebook was that I could create privacy settings so only certain connections or "friends" could see my content, not the entire world.

I looked through Twitter in 2010 but didn't consider using it. It seemed complicated, uninteresting, and even hostile—and I didn't know how to maneuver the features. I also didn't see the need to use it as a social connectivity platform; all "my people" were on Facebook. In 2014, I took a course in social media as part of my master's degree. Getting set up on Twitter was our first assignment and I was overwhelmed. I had no interest in conversing with "strangers" but because this was a graded assignment, I was forced to participate—which changed the trajectory of my career.

After a weekend of digging into the Twitter app and Googling things like "how do I find good hashtags," I felt more comfortable with the platform and how to navigate it, follow other people, and write in a style that fit the short-form posts. After tweeting a few messages with links to articles that I wrote, I quickly learned that the "strangers" I built up as followers were my professional allies. It was more about sharing our unique experiences with each other and gaining insights into what other people in our field were doing, what challenges we were experiencing, and what lessons we learned. And these strangers were nice. They were "my professional people." Some of them even became virtual friends that I still interact with regularly. I've never met them in person, but the digital connection spurred some incredible ideas that we have implemented in our professional work. My curiosity and problem-solving characteristics were activated in the social world of Twitter.

In perfect timing, I met Mona when she started working as Department Chair at Rush University; our offices were right across from each other. We had an immediate connection because I knew she was active on social media. I was in the process of creating an integrated marketing campaign to affect peer ranking scores for our college, and social media was a major component of this reputation-building effort. Mona and I got together and realized very few clinicians and researchers were aware of the benefits of social media, let alone using it to supplement their work and build reputation. So we developed and conducted Twitter workshops and training sessions for them over the next few years. And the rest ... you've read in this book.

What Brought Us Together

Since we connected, we realized there was a great deal of interest from health care professionals to get involved in social media, but they didn't know where to start. Our experiences complemented each other, and we wanted to use our knowledge to address this need in our industry. Our goal is to help you expand your digital presence for yourself, your clinical/research practice, your community, or the world. We have seen how social media has enhanced our own career trajectories and want the same for each of you.

INDEX

Printed in the United States
by Baker & Taylor Publisher Services

Printed in the United States
by Baker & Taylor Publisher Services